OXFORD MEDICAL PUBLICATIONS

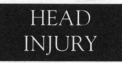

HEAD INJURY

the**facts**

A guide for families and care-givers

thefacts
ALSO AVAILABLE IN THE SERIES

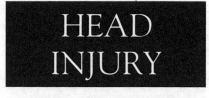

HEAD
INJURY

the**facts**

Second Edition

....

A guide for families and care-givers

....

Dorothy Gronwall,
Philip Wrightson, and Peter Waddel
Auckland Hospital,
Auckland, New Zealand

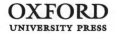

OXFORD
UNIVERSITY PRESS

OXFORD

UNIVERSITY PRESS

Great Clarendon Street, Oxford OX2 6DP

Oxford University Press is a department of the University of Oxford.
It furthers the University's objective of excellence in research, scholarship,
and education by publishing worldwide in

Oxford New York

Auckland Cape Town Dar es Salaam Hong Kong Karachi
Kuala Lumpur Madrid Melbourne Mexico City Nairobi
New Delhi Shanghai Taipei Toronto

With offices in

Argentina Austria Brazil Chile Czech Republic France Greece
Guatemala Hungary Italy Japan South Korea Poland Portugal
Singapore Switzerland Thailand Turkey Ukraine Vietnam

Oxford is a registered trade mark of Oxford University Press
in the UK and in certain other countries

Published in the United States
by Oxford University Press Inc., New York

© Dorothy Gronwall, Philip Wrightson, and Peter Waddell, 1998

The moral rights of the authors have been asserted

Database right Oxford University Press (maker)

First edition published 1990
Second edition 1998
Reprinted 1999, 2002, 2003, 2004, 2005, 2006

A catalogue record for this book is available from the British Library

Library of Congress Cataloging in Publication Data
Gronwall, D. M. A.
Head injury : the facts : a guide for families and care-givers /
Dorothy Gronwall and Philip Wrightson, Peter Waddell.—2nd ed.
(Oxford medical publications) (The facts)
Includes bibliographical references and index.
1. Brain—Wounds and injuries. 2. Brain—Wounds and injuries—
Patients—Rehabilitation. I. Wrightson. Philip. II. Waddell,
Peter. III. Title. IV. Series. V. Series: The facts (Oxford,
England)
[DNLM: 1. Brain injuries—rehabilitation. WL 354 G876h 1997]
RD594.G69 1997 617.4'81044—dc21 97–18414
ISBN 0 19 262713 9 (Pbk)

Printed in Great Britain on acid-free paper by
Clays Ltd, St Ives plc

Foreword to the Second Edition

Jennie Ponsford

It has been seven years since the first edition of *Head Injury: The Facts* was published. No doubt countless head-injured individuals, their families or care-givers, and clinicians have found this book invaluable in guiding them through the various phases of acute care, rehabilitation, community reintegration and adjustment following a head injury. 'The Facts' have not altered. Head injury still causes complex and unique changes, physically, cognitively, and behaviorally, which are exceedingly difficult to grasp, let alone overcome. In spite of technological advances, still no miracle cures have been found.

Unfortunately head-injured people continue to be sent home from emergency departments or admitted to orthopaedic wards with scant attention being paid to the fact that they have sustained a head injury, causing significant stress for the head-injured person, the family, employers, teachers, and others. The case stories recounted in this second edition illustrate a number of common scenarios: the child who is sent back to school without proper assessment or preparation, the lawyer and parent who goes home from the emergency department, unable to cope with a myriad of puzzling symptoms, and the young man with a more severe injury whose limitations are recognized by others, but of which he himself has little awareness or acceptance. In the cases described appropriate methods of assisting these individuals were instituted. However the availability of these kinds of services has improved only a little over the past seven years. With the advent of managed care and emphasis upon economic rationalism we now run the risk of losing the ground that has been gained in service delivery. For this reason it has become even more important that head-injured individuals, their families, and/or care-givers have access to clear, accurate, and balanced information about head injury, and ways if tackling the myriad of physical, cognitive, behavioural, social, and emotional difficulties which may present themselves. There are no easy solutions to any of these problems, but this book provides reassurance that, when properly understood, and given appropriate support or compensatory strategies, difficulties may be overcome, or the injured person can gradually rebuild a life which is meaningful.

Head-injured individuals, their families, and clinicians deserve to benefit from the depth of experience and compassion of these authors.

Foreword to the First Edition

Muriel D. Lezak

This is the book which thoughtful clinicians who work with head-injured patients and the patients' families and friends have been waiting for. It comes from the experiences and concerns of authors who are intensively involved with head-injured patients; as scientists trying to understand the nature of the mental and behavioural disturbances which can follow head injury; as clinicians responsible for evaluating and treating these disturbances; and as care-givers who know well the frustrations, disappointments, confusion, and anxiety which are the everyday lot of so many of these patients and their families.

Until very recently the psychological ramifications of head trauma had been largely overlooked, and they were therefore unknown to almost everybody including the patients and the people close to them. Most people suffering a residual compromise of mental efficiency following an accident with minimal or no loss of consciousness attributed their problems to psychological causes; their physicians often dismissed these patients as neurotics, compensation seekers or both. Misinterpretation of the more profound behavioural and emotional alterations in severely injured people has also been common. Many of these head-injured people have been dismissed by their family, doctors, and themselves as unmotivated and irresponsible, or have ended up in psychiatric facilities carrying one or another – often several – awesome diagnoses. Only patients with obvious crippling or other physical alteration were likely to have the permanent neuropsychological residuals of their brain injuries recognized, although even then higher mental dysfunctions were often ignored or misinterpreted.

As the misdiagnosed patients have suffered from neglect, bewilderment, and despair, families lacking knowledge about their head-injured patient have suffered too. Many families have gone through a progression of torments that begins with puzzlement and then confusion as the patient no longer responds in familiar and appropriate ways. Frustration and anxiety arise as the uninformed family members discover that their efforts are ineffective, and may even make the situation worse. Many family members feel shame and guilt at what they believe are their failures to cope with the patient's problem behaviours.

Depression is almost inevitable. Disruption of once solid family relationships is not an infrequent occurrence which further compounds their misery.

It has only been in recent years, as the vicissitudes of head-trauma victims have become known, that there has been a dawning awareness of the profound interdependence between head-injured patients and their families: how the patient can affect the family, what the family can do for the patient. Until now, this information has not been generally available. *Head Injury: The Facts* provides the information family members need, for their own well-being and that of the head-injured patient, by taking the reader from the patient's arrival in an emergency room through typical hospital and post-hospital experiences, emphasizing all the while what the family should know and what family members can do at each stage of the patient's course. More than a manual for patients' families, this book should be required reading for every professional who works with head-injured patients to ensure that they have a practical appreciation of their patients' behaviour and emotions, and sensitivity to the feelings and needs of their patients' families.

Acknowledgements

We are grateful for the support of the Medical Research Council of New Zealand and of the New Zealand Neurological Foundation in funding the research of the two senior authors into the effects of head injury. We are also grateful to all families and all the head-injured people we have worked with over the years for allowing us to learn from them and for giving us the insight that we needed in order to go some way towards understanding how head injury affected you all. Many of you will recognize yourselves in this book. Without you it could never have been written.

Preface

The first edition of this book was written to try to answer the many questions that parents, spouses, and friends wanted to know about head injury and it's effects. It has been very rewarding to get feed-back from people in many parts of the world that the book has indeed been of some help. This second edition updates some of the information, and fine-tunes some of the earlier account, but basically the effects of head injury are the same, whether the accident occurred at the time the book was first published, or in 1998, when this second edition is printed.

There are still no magic cures. Head injury can be, and often is, a long-term, twenty-four hours a day, seven days a week problem. While the problem obviously affects the person who has had the injury most directly, the lives of many, many other people are touched. We hope this book will help friends, families, employers, and school-teachers, among others, to understand some of the complexities of head injury, and some of the reasons why the head-injured person cannot always be expected to cope as well as he had done before his injury.

This other impetus for writing the book was the paucity of rehabilitation facilities for survivors of head trauma. In 1990 our preface concluded with the following paragraph:

> The tragic lack of appropriate rehabilitation facilities for survivors of head trauma is unfortunately seen all over the world. There are some signs that this is changing, and this change has come about because of the demands of concerned families. We hope that this book will assist you to bring about the changes that you need.

Sadly, seven years later, head injury rehabilitation is still a Cinderella service. Where advances have been made, these have mostly been driven by concerned families and concerned clinicians. We need to work together, armed with the facts about head injury, to persuade the holders of the health and rehabilitation purse strings that it is not cost-effective to spend thousands of dollars on saving someone's life after a head-injury accident, and then to cut off the support that world allow them to achieve their economic potential, and gain an optimum quality of life.

Auckland, New Zealand   D. G.
October 1997   P. W.
                                                                 P. W.

the**facts**

CONTENTS

Contents

1
Introduction

In recent years the road toll has tended to edge downward in developed countries perhaps because of an increasing awareness of the need to build safety features into motor vehicles, and perhaps due to an improvement in the education of drivers and law enforcers. The hidden road toll, the effect on the drivers, passengers, and pedestrians who suffer head injuries in traffic accidents, has also edged downward. Unfortunately there is still a horrendously high number of head injuries overall. People are still head injured in falls, in sports, particularly contact sports, in industry, and in violence on the streets. Young men still make up the majority of these cases, with small children and the elderly also at risk.

In many countries there has been a change from hospital-based to community care, so that fewer head-injured people are now admitted to hospital and more are treated only in casualty departments or by their own family doctor. A recent survey in North America found that when all these cases were included, more than 600 people out of every 100 000 received a head injury each year. There is also increasing awareness that problems are not limited to people who receive a head injury severe enough for them to be treated in hospital. Indeed in the United States it has been shown that people who had not been admitted to hospital after the accident make up half of all the days off work and school which are missed due to head injury.

However appalling this figure is, though, it is still only part of the picture. For each new head-injury case there are many other people affected. Family and friends, employers and work-mates, and even casual acquaintances have their lives touched by head-injury accidents. In the main, though, head injury is a family affair.

This book has been written for families who have a head-injured member, for people with an injured partner or an injured friend, and especially for all those who, because of circumstances, have taken on the role of care-givers. We have not addressed the book directly to the person who has had the head injury, because the injury may have affected the ability to cope with working through it. Concentration is invariably impaired following head injury, as is the ability to remember new material. However, we hope that those who have made sufficient recovery from their accident to read this will find that the information which we have given helps them to understand the injury and its effects. Except where we are specifically talking about women we have referred to the head injury person as 'he' for convenience because most head injury cases are male.

Over the past decade or two there has been a surge of interest in the problem of head injury. Improved medical techniques have meant that many more people are surviving injuries which in the past would have been fatal. Many articles have been written about the effects of head injury and its treatment but most of the articles are by professionals and written for professionals. The articles appear in scientific journals which are not easily accessible, and which may not be helpful to you in any case. Yet families desperately want to know and understand what has happened when one of them suffers a head injury. Time and again, before the first edition of this book was published, as professionals working in the field of head-injury rehabilitation we had been asked by families and friends where they could find a book to explain about the head injury. The book was designed as a source of information which would be comprehensive but not too medical or technical. We hope this new edition continues to satisfy this need.

How this book is organized

The next chapter looks at the mechanics of head injury and explains how particular parts of the brain become damaged. Chapter 3 covers the time in hospital. The different kinds of hospital treatment and procedures are described, and the sort of information these techniques can and cannot give is explained. Chapter 3 also describes the roles of different members of the hospital staff and what part each plays in the treatment of the head-injured person.

The remaining chapters talk about the period after he leaves hospital. Head injury is usually a long-term problem, and the emphasis which this book puts on the time after the spell in hospital reflects this. Many of the problems that result from a head injury often only become evident after the head-injured person leaves hospital.

Chapter 4 discusses the practical issues of the post-hospital period. Where will he go? Who will look after him? What treatment will he get, and where? Family involvement and support is a big help to him during the time in hospital. After leaving hospital family involvement and support becomes vital. Usually families are enthusiastic and want to do as much as they can to help, but often, because they are not aware of what is available, many do not ask for the assistance which they could get. Chapter 4 points out the importance of getting the financial and other assistance which you are entitled to. Coping with the care of a head-injured person can be a long-term full-time job. Trying to cope with the extra chores that must be done, and with the extra expense that will be involved on an income that is often reduced because of his accident, makes this job even more difficult.

Chapter 5 is the largest and probably the most important in the book. This chapter covers the effect of head injury on emotions and thinking, on how the head-injured person behaves. Most people, even those with apparently minor injuries, can have some or all of the problems that are described. This chapter is relevant to everyone, regardless of the type of accident their friend, relative, or partner has had.

Chapter 6 is rather different, covering some special problems that only a proportion of people will have. Some people, for a while, are paralyzed down one side of their body after a head injury. Some have difficulty understanding what is said to them, or have trouble talking. Some may have fits or blackouts. Chapter 6 explains why these things happen, and what families can do to cope with them.

Chapter 7 describes the special problems faced by different age groups. It also covers the different (and difficult) problems that head injury can cause when the accident victim is a parent or a partner. Although most head-injured cases are young adult males, accidents can happen to anyone and at any age. The effects of head injury will be similar regardless of the age at which it happens, but these effects pose different problems when they happen at different stages of life. In the first few years of infancy and early childhood, for example, an enormous amount of learning needs to take place. To learn well you must have a memory that works well, but head injury almost invariably interferes with how well the memory system will work. So an infant who has an accident when he or she is two may take longer to reach some developmental milestones.

Chapter 8 deals with the subject of how long the problems will last. One of the most frustrating things that families have to face is not being able to plan for the future. How long will it be before the head-injured person is able to look after himself again? Will he ever get back to the life he had before the accident? Should his mother give up the career that she may have carved for herself after her children grew up? Should she take leave of absence? You will not find the answers to these questions in this chapter but we hope that you will understand why they are such difficult questions to answer.

Even if no one can tell you exactly how long it will be before your head-injured relative will be well enough to think about going back to work or to school, in most cases the time will come eventually. Chapter 9 talks about this time, and how the change should be made. It is very important that employers or teachers understand that the person who has had a head injury will get tired more quickly and that he will be more easily distracted. This chapter is therefore addressed to employers and teachers as well as the people closely involved in caring for him. However, it is important to remember that family support is equally if not more necessary during the gradual shift back to work.

A few head-injured people will never resume employment, and Chapter 10 examines the long-term adjustments that they and their families have to make. There are many sorts of loss after severe head injury. There are the obvious losses of physical and mental functions, and the loss of self-esteem and of independence which result. There are the losses of relationships and social life, as well as the loss of careers. Chapter 10 discusses these losses, and suggests how families and head-injured persons can cope with adjusting to permanent disability.

Chapter 11 looks at the future, at the resources which, in an ideal world, should be provided for the head-injured person. It is aimed at those who have the responsibility for the management of the head-injured person, and suggests some steps which can be taken to make sure that these services are provided. This chapter was written in 1990 for the first edition. Sadly there is still the gap between the standard of acute care, which is generally excellent, and that of rehabilitation services, which tends to be very patchy.

At the end of this book there are some suggestions for further reading, and finally, we have included two appendices. Appendix A is an explanation of many of the technical terms that are used when talking about head injury. Not all these terms have been used in this book but they are likely to come up when you are talking with doctors or rehabilitation therapists. This appendix should help you make sense of what has been said or written. Appendix B gives contact addresses of organizations which have been set up to provide support for people who have a relative or friend who has been involved in a head-injury accident. There are three sections in this appendix; for Australasia, for the United Kingdom, and for North America. We believe that it will be helpful for you to have the addresses of contact agencies for overseas countries as well as for your own, as there may be cases where a friend or relative has the head injury away from home.

How to use this book

We have aimed to make it as easy as possible for you to find information about any particular problem as it arises. You will find headings in the chapters, and the page numbers of each of these headings are shown in the contents. You may be reading this book for the first time while you are sitting beside your relative in Critical Care, or you may be reading it for the first time many months after the accident. In either case you will be asking for solutions, or at least explanations. The headings are designed to allow you to get directly to the information that you need, now, when you need it. We know, because the caregivers that we have worked with over the years have told us so, that you will want to know everything that you can about head injury. We suspect that you may read this book right through at first, even though, at any one time, some of the sections will not apply in your case.

Case histories

As in the first edition of this book we have included three case histories to illustrate and summarize many of the points that we cover. For this edition we have selected three different people's stories to help you understand head injuries. These cases are introduced below. Note that names and personal details have been changed to protect the identity of the patients.

Samuel — aged 11 years

Samuel was keen to get home on the day of his accident. It was his birthday and he had been given a pair of roller blades by his parents, but they would not let him take them to school. The first thing he did, even before having his usual huge afternoon snack, was to try them out in the carport. This was a bit tame, so he decided to take on the drive, which had a nice slope right down to the road. He flew faster and faster, but could not stop when he reached the road, tripped on the kerb, and ended up on the opposite footpath with one leg doubled up beneath him.

Samuel was the youngest of a family of four, had a reputation as a dare-devil, and excelled at sports. However, he was not academic, and only tolerated the classroom as something he had to put up with between sports and games. He was two years behind his age in reading, and for some time his parents had been considering getting him some help with mathematics.

We shall meet Samuel again in Chapters 4, 5, 6, 7, 8 and 9.

Jonas — aged 20 years

Jonas is an apprentice carpenter who ran his car into the back of a stationary truck on the way home from a Friday night drink with the boys after work. This drink had turned into several, and his mates had tried to persuade him to come with them in their taxi, but he would not leave his prized car in the inner-city hotel car park. He was in the final year of his apprenticeship, with only 600 hours to go before he had completed his time.

He had recently moved into a flat with three others, as he was frustrated by the restrictions his parents placed on him at home. They were worried about his heavy drinking and would not let him have parties or invite his mates round. They also objected to the continual oil marks on the concrete drive after he had been working on his car.

We shall meet Jonas again in Chapters 3, 4, 5, 6, 7, 8 and 9.

Pauline — aged 42 years

Pauline was one of those people who managed to juggle marriage and children and a successful and demanding career. Her head injury happened completely by accident. She was walking from her office to the law court to a fascinating case where she was confident the defendant was not guilty and she hoped she would be able to get an early acquittal. She was reviewing the evidence in her mind as she hurried along the street when the load on a delivery truck came adrift, and a large carton hit her on the shoulder and knocked her to the ground. She hit her head when she fell and lost consciousness immediately.

At the time of her accident she had two children aged 14 and 16, and a supportive husband who enjoyed preparing the evening meal when he got home after his work as a secondary school teacher.

We shall meet Pauline again in Chapters 4, 5, 6, 7, 8 and 9.

2 What happens in a head injury

In this chapter we will try to explain the ways in which the brain may be damaged in an accident, and the effects that this damage can cause. We have found that most families and injured people want to know more about this, and that it seems to help them both in the early days after the accident and in dealing with the problems that come later. You should remember that we are describing a wide range of possibilities, and that the person that you are concerned with may have been affected in only one or two of the ways we will be talking about. If you are in doubt about anything, or if what we say worries you, talk it over with the doctor who has been your contact at the hospital or clinic, or with your family doctor.

The sorts of head injury

A head injury sets off a train of events. It can help to think of these in three stages, beginning with the 'first injury', the direct effect of the accident. After this, in the next hour or two, the 'second injury', can follow, and in the next day or two the 'third injury'. Each of these injuries can have a decisive effect on the quality of recovery and the success of rehabilitation.

The 'first injury'

Three sorts of first injury
Closed
Open — penetrating
Crushing

Closed head injury

The commonest way the brain can be injured is by 'acceleration', which usually produces a 'closed head injury'. It is called this because there does not need to be a break of the skin or an open wound. This happens when the head suddenly changes its motion. Examples are the sudden stop when a car runs into a brick wall (deceleration) or when you are jerked forward when you have stopped at a traffic light and another car runs into yours from behind (acceleration). Another example is the sudden roll of the head with a knock-out punch to the jaw (rotation).

As the head is accelerated, decelerated or rotated the brain is forced to follow the movements of the skull, and as it is soft and jelly-like it gets twisted in the process. The brain is made up from billions of nerve fibres that run from one part of the brain to another, and as the twisting occurs these fibres are stretched and damaged. Even quite mild injuries of this sort can have serious consequences if they affect important and sensitive areas of the brain.

The arteries and veins which run through the brain can also be damaged. They may leak fluid out into the brain so that it swells, or they can be torn right across so that blood runs out, making a bruise which is very like one in any other part of the body.

Also, because there is room for the brain to move a little inside the skull, with the acceleration it slides on the inner surface of the bone. This surface has ridges and sharp edges which bump and bruise the surface of the brain, causing yet more damage.

Open or penetrating head injury

Another sort of 'first injury' is the 'open' or 'penetrating' injury. In this type of injury the scalp is cut through, the bone beneath it is broken through and the brain underneath is damaged and perhaps left exposed. The causes of this sort of injury range from falling on the sharp edge of a stone curb, through flying through a car windscreen to being hit by a bullet. Sometimes the injury can be quite localized and the brain away from the immediate area may be undamaged, so that in the long term there may be little disability in spite of what at the time looked like a very frightening injury. Unfortunately open injuries often occur together with an acceleration type injury, and it is usually the acceleration injury that determines the outcome.

Crushing head injury

The least common type of 'first injury' is the 'crushing injury': the head may be caught between a boat and the wharf or under the wheel of a car. Often the important damage is not to the brain itself but to the base of the skull and the nerves that run out through it, and there may be no loss of consciousness.

In all types of 'first injury' almost every time what really matters is the injury to the brain itself. The scalp can be torn and the bone of the skull can be broken or parts of it lost, but if there is any long-term disability it will be because of damage to the brain underneath.

The second accident

Many serious injuries result from high speed car accidents. The head is damaged when the first collision occurs, but then the victim may be flung out of the car and strike their head again, perhaps even several times, and also incur other injuries. This is a very important cause of multiple major injuries, and it must be emphasized that efficient seat belts will stop this happening.

The 'first injury' — occurs in the first 2 seconds
Brain accelerated, decelerated or rotated
Nerve fibres stretched
Arteries and veins torn
With or without an open wound

Note: Sometimes there is a second accident
        Seatbelts stop the second accident

The 'first injury' to the brain as we have described it takes place within a second. In this short time much of the fate of the victim is decided. Not all of it, however, because in many people there are at least two further 'injuries'.

The 'second injury'

Many accidents happen in the worst surroundings: at night, in the rain, away from expert help. The injured person can be crushed into the twisted body of his car, with his face buried in the dashboard. His breathing is often blocked with vomited food, or by blood from an injury to the nose or face. Air cannot get to the lungs, so that the amount of oxygen in the blood becomes much less than it should be. The brain becomes starved of oxygen, killing its cells and adding to the damage from the first injury.

Injuries to other parts of the body are common in road accidents like this, and often a great deal of blood is lost. This lowers the blood pressure below safe limits, reduces the supply of blood to the brain and so makes the brain damage worse.

Understanding this chain of events has led to great improvements in the way in which ambulance and rescue services operate. The first thing that they do at the scene of the accident is to make sure that breathing is free and easy. Probably they will then set up an urgent transfusion to replace the blood that has been lost and to bring the blood pressure up to safe levels. In this way the brain is protected during the journey to hospital.

The 'second injury' — occurs in the first hour
Obstructed breathing deprives brain of oxygen
Blood loss lowers blood pressure and reduces supply of blood and
  oxygen to the brain

The 'third injury'

The injuries that we have described up to now have occurred in the first second after the accident and in the first hour or so. The 'third injury' can occur any time after this, usually in the next 24–48 hours, occasionally up to a month or two later. There are several forms it can take.

Bruising and swelling of the brain

When it is damaged at the first impact the brain reacts to the injury in the same way as the rest of the body does, by bruising; body fluids and blood leak out into it and it swells. However, the effect is more important than in other parts of the body, because the brain is enclosed in the unyielding skull. Even slight swelling squeezes the brain, so that blood has difficulty in circulating through it. In severe cases the pressure in the brain rises to the point that the blood circulation stops entirely, and the brain then dies.

The pressure inside the skull (you may hear it called the 'intra-cranial pressure' or 'ICP') is therefore something of great importance.

The medical team needs to know what it is when they are planning treatment, and much of what they do will be designed to keep it at a safe level. As we will see in Chapter 3, sometimes intracranial pressure is measured continuously and displayed on one of the 'monitor' screens around the patient in intensive care.

To keep the intracranial pressure down the brain swelling must be kept to a minimum. To do this, the first thing is to make sure that the blood coming to the brain has plenty of oxygen in it and that it is removing waste products like carbon dioxide. The blood pressure must be kept high enough to keep the brain circulation going. Air — usually with oxygen added — must flow in and out of the lungs without obstruction. There must be no coughing or straining, which would put the intracranial pressure up and start fresh bleeding in damaged areas of the brain. Finally, the amount of water and salt in the body must be kept at the right level to reduce the flow of tissue fluid into the brain. Blood tests will be done frequently to make sure of this, and the amount of fluids given will be strictly controlled.

Blood clots

We have described how at the time of the original injury small veins and arteries were torn and that this results in bruising of the brain. Sometimes larger blood vessels are torn, so that enough blood escapes at one place to form a ball of blood clot which compresses and damages the brain around it. It also increases the intracranial pressure, and if the bleeding does not stop it can push the pressure over the limit at which it becomes fatal.

These clots are not very common, but they are important. They sometimes occur after quite minor injuries, even when the person has been knocked out for only a short period and has apparently recovered. This is one of the reasons why even minor injuries are taken seriously by hospital accident departments, and why people are kept under observation until the risk of a clot forming is likely to be over. When there is a serious injury the risk is much greater, and many of the observations made in intensive care are designed to detect them as early as possible. The other reason why blood clots are so important is that if they do occur, they can usually be treated successfully by operation.

In discussing the situation with the family the medical team may say where the clot is; it could be within the brain itself (an intra-cerebral clot), between the brain and the dura, the thick membrane that surrounds the brain and separates it from the bone of the skull (a subdural clot), or between the dura and the bone (an extradural clot). The exact location really only matters to the surgeon who removes it, and it is probably better not to be concerned about the detail.

There is, however, one special case that you should know about, the 'chronic subdural haematoma'. This is more often seen in older people and can follow quite a minor injury. What happens is that a small clot forms between the brain and the dura, not big enough to be detected at first. This slowly grows in size over a number of weeks until it is large enough to cause symptoms. Fortunately it can usually be removed by a simple operation, with effective results.

Another condition which comes on later with symptoms rather like those of the chronic subdural haematoma is 'post-traumatic hydrocephalus'. This occurs when the circulation of fluid round the brain is blocked by the scarring which follows the brain injury. The fluid accumulates inside the brain and the intracranial pressure rises. Again this complication can be treated very effectively by a small operation.

The 'third injury'
A *day or more later*:
brain bruising and swelling
blood clots

A *week or more later*:
chronic subdural haematoma
post-traumatic hydrocephalus

Damage to the skull

It was said earlier that it was the damage to the brain itself that was the most important thing about a head injury. This is so, but the skull is often damaged as well and sometimes needs treatment.

Fractures of the vault

The commonest damage, a 'linear fracture', is a crack in the vault of the skull, the rounded dome of the head. This is usually not more than a millimeter or so wide and is not of itself important. It does of course mean that the blow to the head was quite severe. Some of the complications we have mentioned are more likely to occur and the patient will probably be watched more closely. The fracture heals quickly, usually with scar tissue rather than bone, and leaves no weakness.

A blow to the vault of the skull can crack the bone and dent it, sometimes pushing a piece of bone far enough in to damage the underlying brain. This 'depressed fracture' may need an operation, not usually a serious one, to replace the fragments of bone and to deal with any damaged brain underneath.

Fractures of the base of the skull

When the injury has been particularly severe the bones of the base of the skull may be broken. Damage to the cerebellum and to the inner ear is likely, causing problems later with balance and vertigo, as well as an increased risk of other complications because of the violence of the injury.

Fractures of the forehead, nose, and eye sockets

A fracture which involves the bone of the forehead or the nose may result in a hole in the roof of the nose which communicates with the space round the brain. Brain fluid (cerebrospinal fluid) may leak out and drip from the nose and, more important, bacteria may get in through the hole and infect the brain, causing meningitis. If there is a leak, in the short term infection can be prevented by antibiotics, but unless the leak stops soon of its own accord an operation will be needed to block up the hole and make a permanent repair. This can usually be done safely and effectively. A leak of the same sort can occur when there is a fracture which involves the bone around the middle ear; this usually heals of its own accord.

Some severe injuries fracture the bone of the eye sockets and the middle part of the face, as well as the vault of the skull. This can affect proper eye movement, the nasal sinuses and the alignment of the teeth of the upper jaw. An operation, usually by a team of neurosurgeons and plastic surgeons, may be needed to correct the deformity.

Fractures with open wounds

When there is an 'open' or 'penetrating' injury the bone of the skull is likely to be damaged. Urgent operation will be needed to clean the wound and get rid of infection, and to close the skin. Sometimes pieces of bone will be missing, or too badly damaged to replace. This is not important at the time, the wound can be safely closed and no harm will result. Later, if the gap in the skull is big enough to be a risk, or if it is too disfiguring, it can be filled in. After several months, when the wound has healed and all chance of infection has gone, a bone graft or a plastic or metal plate can be put in to close the hole.

Damage to the skull

Fractures of the vault:

linear fractures: only important because they show there has been a significant injury

depressed fractures: bone may need to be lifted back into place

Fractures of the forehead, nose, and eye sockets:

may cause leaks of cerebrospinal fluid

ugly deformities may need operation

Fractures with wounds:

need operation to prevent infection and close wound

gaps in the skull may need to be filled in

Late effects of head injury

Multiple head injuries

Many people have more than one head injury. This is very important for two reasons. First, after one injury the brain may become abnormally sensitive. If there is another accident within a week or two of the first one, while the brain is still recovering, there may be a reaction quite out of proportion to the severity of either of the injuries. Within an hour massive brain swelling can occur, often with a fatal result. This is an important reason why sportsmen who have been concussed should not be allowed to play again until they have fully recovered, preferably allowing at least three weeks for this.

Secondly, when there have been several head injuries there is often a general loss of brain capacity. Even if there has been only one injury, a second one seems to have much more of an effect than would be expected, and after each further injury the disturbance becomes more marked. This progressive damage can occur with quite minor injuries. Football players after only three or four concussions can begin to show a deterioration in their thinking powers. An extreme example is the punch-drunk boxer; he does not need to have been knocked out often, a sufficient number of head punches without this are enough to do the damage.

The reason for this progressive deterioration is probably that each injury kills some nerve cells, so that the total number available to do the work of the brain is steadily reduced. Eventually the reserve which we all have is used up. With further injury, and sometimes with the loss of brain cells that occurs with age, there is not enough brain left to do the work asked of it and obvious symptoms appear.

Multiple head injuries
Some brain function is lost with each injury
Brain loss adds up with multiple minor injuries
Blows without loss of consciousness can destroy brain cells

Post-traumatic epilepsy

When the brain is damaged it heals with a scar. As it does this the brain around the damaged area may begin to work in an abnormal way. It can become irritable and unstable and liable to bursts of uncontrolled activity. The disturbance tends to spread wide of the damaged area and involve the rest of the brain, and this produces an epileptic fit. This occurs most often after a severe injury, especially when there has been much bruising or bleeding into the brain, or if there has been an open wound. It can sometimes happen after a minor injury if there has been a small bruise in a particularly sensitive area.

The effect of the injury on brain function

It has been known for a long time that when particular areas of the brain are damaged there are characteristic effects on its function. For instance, damage to the side of the brain half way from the front to the back (the 'parietal' area) results in weakness of the arm or leg on the opposite side of the body. Damage on the left side tends to impair speech. Injury to the brain behind the forehead (the 'frontal' area) results in changes in behaviour, and loss of self restraint and insight (for diagram showing areas of the brain see the end of Appendix A.).

When there is a localized injury to the brain, perhaps caused by an open wound or a penetrating injury, only one of these functions may be affected. Most head injuries, however, are closed injuries caused by acceleration, with multiple areas of the brain damaged. Some or perhaps many of the brain functions may be affected, some more severely than others. Again, while wounds or penetrating injuries usually damage just the surface of the brain, in closed injuries the nerve fibres deep in the brain are affected. These include the central parts of the brain which are vital for keeping us alert, and it is the damage here that results in the most typical symptom of head injury — coma.

Often torn in the deeper and more severe injuries are the bundles of nerves which run down from the surface of the brain to the 'brain stem' and spinal cord. These normally control movement and sensation and their damage results in a characteristic type of paralysis of the arms and legs, sometimes seen in the early stages of recovery from a severe injury. The legs are stretched out straight and stiff, and the arms are bent up at the elbow, a rigid 'spastic' paralysis. Both legs are usually affected, and only one arm. When movement eventually returns, it is likely to be awkward and uncoordinated.

The movements of the throat are under the control of the brain stem and after a serious injury of this sort speech and swallowing are often impaired. The brain stem is also responsible for body functions which are not under conscious control, such as breathing, heart beat and blood pressure, and body temperature, and upset of these functions may be one of the factors which determine survival in the early days after the injury.

Some of the results we have described above will be evident while the victim is still unconscious or semi-conscious. It will not be until later that the more subtle effects on thinking and personality become obvious. These will be partly due to damage to the special areas of the brain we mentioned before, and in the more serious injuries to the widespread tearing of nerve fibres that affects all the working parts of the brain.

Effects on brain function
Visible effects:
coma
loss of power in limbs (often spastic)
impaired speech and swallowing

Hidden effects:
on heart, blood pressure, and breathing (in the early stages)
on thinking and personality (in the later stages)

Recovery after injury

Although it is not known for certain, it is likely that most of the brain cells which have been damaged will not get back to useful work. The majority of improvement that is seen after a head injury is due to re-organization of the brain which is undamaged. Using the large reserves of brain function that we all have, intact areas take over from those that are no longer functional. Obviously if these reserves of brain have been reduced by previous injuries, or by the natural loss of nerve cells with age, recovery will be less complete.

Recovery of function is therefore a matter of learning and re-education. It may take a long time, comparable to the years spent in school. Success will depend on consistent teaching and patient encouragement, and must take each person's abilities and problems into account. It must also be realistic, and not set goals which are out of reach. This is the basis on which the programme of rehabilitation needs to be planned.

Recovery after injury
The best use must be made of undamaged abilities
Re-education can take as long as education
Rehabilitation is a full-time job

Failure to recover

Sometimes after a severe injury recovery ceases before there has been a return of consciousness or any meaningful response. It is possible for the person to continue for months or even years without change. This condition, sometimes called the persistent vegetative state, poses immense problems both for the families and for the institutions caring for the patient. Occasional recoveries after years in the condition make it difficult to be completely certain that the outlook is hopeless. Even if one could be sure that the outlook was indeed hopeless, withdrawal of life support is still a terrible decision to make. However, recent research into the condition has produced some guidelines which can help and support families faced with these decisions, and the legal situation has become clearer.

Brain death

It is sometimes not possible to overcome the effects of injury. The cause is almost always that it has been impossible to control the swelling of the brain and the pressure inside the skull. As the pressure rises, the circulation of blood through the brain slows and eventually stops. After a few minutes the brain is irreparably damaged. The spinal cord, being outside the skull, may remain alive for a while, and there may be some automatic reflex movements of the limbs, but all other functions stop. Although it is usually only too obvious when brain death has taken place, because of the need to be absolutely certain the medical staff will follow a routine of tests, repeated several times at intervals of an hour or two. The crucial results are that there are no reflex responses that require brain function. The pupils of the eyes are widely dilated and do not react to light. There is no effort to breathe even with the maximum stimulation. Other tests may be used to confirm the findings. The electroencephalogram, which records the electrical activity of the brain, will be silent. X-ray tests can confirm that there is no circulation of blood to the brain.

When it is certain that there is no longer any chance of recovery of function of the brain, it is usually taken that there is no use in continuing treatment, and if the family agrees the life-support systems can be withdrawn. If it has been decided that treatment should stop, the family may be asked for their agreement to allow body organs such as the heart or kidneys to be removed for use as transplants. It is very difficult for the family to make decisions at a time like this. There may be good reasons to say no. However, it is worthwhile here to reassure you about two questions which are sometimes asked. Firstly, there is no question of taking these organs unless there is absolutely no doubt that there has been brain death. It will not be done until the tests described above have been done and checked, and until an independent medical team is absolutely certain about them. Secondly, you might be uncertain whether the transplants really do good. About this there is no doubt whatever; they will probably mean the difference between life and death for two or more people.

3
In hospital

The care of someone with a head injury starts with first aid at the site of the accident, continues with rescue by the paramedics and ambulance, and is followed through by a team working in the hospital, using a wide range of facilities.

Whether you are the patient or one of the family, if you have not been involved with a hospital before you may feel very lost and frightened by this large organization, with all its power and prestige. It is a good idea, therefore, to know how a hospital works, who you may meet and what they do. It is also a good idea to remember that you have very definite rights in this situation, and that the whole of this organization has been set up for your benefit.

To give you the best idea of how it all works we will follow Jonas, the young man introduced in Chapter 1 who has had a serious traffic accident, from the crash site to the time that he leaves hospital. After this we will talk about people with less serious injuries and discuss some other special situations.

Rescue: first aid and the ambulance

Jonas was on his way home after Friday night drinks with his workmates when he drove his car at high speed into the back of a parked truck. His head broke the windscreen, he was knocked unconscious and there were deep cuts on his face and scalp from the broken glass. Another car was behind him when the accident occurred. Fortunately the driver had a cell-phone and could call for an ambulance, but it was still 15 minutes before it could reach them.

In Chapter 2 we called this 15 minutes the time of the 'second injury'. The patient may be unable to breathe properly because of the position he is lying in, or because his throat is blocked with blood or vomit. The injured brain does not get enough oxygen, causing further damage. The motorist who came to his aid tried to get Jonas's face and mouth clear of vomited beer and blood as best he could, but at the same time he had to be careful not to move him too much in case there were neck or other injuries. As an aside, even if you have been sensible and have taken first aid classes, in real life situations it is not so easy, and you should not feel guilty if you cannot cope as well as you would like.

When the ambulance arrived, it was staffed by paramedics who were expert in dealing with severe injuries. They started by making sure he could breathe easily. His mouth and throat were full of vomit and his air passages were partly blocked, so they put a tube down Jonas's throat into the windpipe to make sure that the airway was unobstructed. A collar was placed round his neck to stabilize it in case there was a fracture. Dressings were put on his scalp and face wounds to control the bleeding.

An important factor in the 'second injury' is loss of blood. If there is severe bruising or a wound which bleeds heavily the blood pressure will fall and the injured brain will be starved of the oxygen it needs. Therefore the paramedics put up a transfusion to replace the large amount of blood which Jonas had lost, and were able to bring the blood pressure up to a level at which the ride to hospital would be safe. As blood itself needs cross matching in the laboratory before it can be given, at the site of an accident blood substitutes are used.

Jonas needed to be in hospital as soon as possible. Helicopters can cut the travelling time down and are most often used when the accident has occurred a long way from hospital, in rough country or away from roads. The accommodation for the patient and paramedics can be cramped and though a road ambulance may take a little longer on the journey it may be easier to keep a close watch on the patient.

Paramedics at the scene of the accident will:
Ensure that the victim is breathing freely
Replace lost blood
Make wounds and fractures safe for transport

Reaching hospital

As soon as Jonas reached hospital the medical team made a complete examination. It was obvious that he was deeply unconscious. In spite of the tube that was inserted by the paramedics he was still not breathing easily. The mouth and throat were cleaned and a new tube (an 'endotracheal' tube) was threaded through his nose and into his windpipe to give him a clear airway. This was then connected to a mechanical ventilator to do his breathing for him. Jonas was then given muscle relaxing drugs to let him rest quietly without coughing or straining, both of which are bad for the brain. When this had been done oxygen could get to his blood, his colour became better and it was obvious that his general condition had improved.

The rest of his body was then examined, starting with the head and looking particularly for injuries to the neck, chest, abdomen and spine, all areas which are often injured in this sort of accident. X-rays of the chest and neck were done as a routine. Fortunately in Jonas's case there was no sign of damage. The amount of blood that had been lost was assessed. It was more than what could be safely replaced with blood substitutes, so blood was cross-matched and a transfusion started.

Essential checks on arrival at hospital
Breathing checked
Blood loss assessed
Head injury status checked
Neck, spine, chest, abdomen, and limbs checked

All this initial assessment and treatment was done at a run, and was completed within 15 minutes of Jonas being wheeled through the door. Notice that so far there has been little detail of the head injury. This may be surprising, but in fact at this stage the only thing that needs to be done for the head injury is to give the brain the best conditions to recover — a good circulation, plenty of oxygen, and no straining.

Now that the first assessment has been done, it is the time for the head injury to be examined in more detail. When Jonas first came into hospital and before the muscle relaxing drugs were given, a rapid examination of brain function was made. The depth of unconsciousness was recorded as a 'coma score', so that changes with time could be followed. His arms and legs were examined to see if they moved when the skin was pinched, and the pupils of the eyes were tested to see how they reacted to light. A note was made of the wounds to his scalp and face and of the bruises on the head, which can give useful clues to the damage inside. The amount of information that can be obtained from an unconscious patient is limited, but these simple tests will give a useful idea of how much damage there has been to the brain.

Jonas was lucky because when he was first examined all four limbs moved equally and his pupils reacted normally to light. This suggested that at least at this stage there was no gross damage to his brain. However, in the next hour or two he would enter the stage where the chance of a 'third injury' that we talked about in Chapter 2 became important. If Jonas had not been so badly injured and if he had remained partially awake the development of this complication would have been shown by his becoming less conscious and perhaps by one side of the body becoming weak or paralysed. Because Jonas was deeply unconscious and because he had been given relaxing drugs which abolished movement, these signs were not available. The team therefore had to rely on high-technology tests, and as soon as possible X-rays were taken of his head.

High-technology tests

X-rays

Ordinary X-rays show only the bone of the skull, not the brain. It is of course important to know whether there is a fracture of the skull, or if any fragments of bone have been pushed into the brain, but at this stage what matters is what is happening to the brain itself. The state of the bone is only a rough guide to this. To show up the brain itself, special methods are needed.

CT scan

The CT ('Computerized Tomographic') scanner uses X-rays to show the soft tissue of the brain itself. It can be seen if the brain is bruised or swollen and whether a blood clot has formed.

MR scan

The MR ('nuclear Magnetic Resonance') scanner does not use X-rays but a combination of radio waves and a very strong magnetic field. It is very effective at showing up the condition of the brain itself.

Emergency Departments in most larger hospitals have access to CT scanners, and they are a rapid and reliable guide to treatment. MR scanners are less likely to be available. They are as effective as CT for emergency work, and more informative in less urgent brain disease. However, they are slower than CT and the very strong magnetic fields that they use make it difficult to use ordinary respirators and monitoring equipment when an unconscious patient is being examined.

Jonas was taken to the CT scanner with his transfusion lines and ventilator attached. The examination showed that there was in fact a clot of blood of considerable size between the bone of the skull and the outer covering of the brain (the 'dura mater') just above his right ear, with much pressure on the brain. This had to be removed, and an urgent neurosurgical operation was needed.

Clues to what is happening in the brain

CT scans: give the most complete picture

Skull X-rays
Bruises, wounds } provide some information

Depth of coma
Movement } provide information only when no muscle relaxing drugs are used

---

The people involved up to now

The team that has worked on Jonas up to now is called the Intensive Care team, sometimes the Critical Care or the Trauma team. They are the experts in dealing with severely injured people whose need is to be kept alive and protected from the effects of their multiple injuries. When problems arise in special fields the Intensive Care team will call on other experts: orthopaedic (bone and joint) surgeons for fractures, abdominal or chest surgeons for injuries to the trunk, and neurosurgeons for the head.

One of the team rang Jonas's family as soon as the ambulance brought him in, and then talked with them as soon as they arrived at the Accident Department. He told them that Jonas's injuries were serious, and that they would have to prepare themselves for the possibility that he might not survive. At this stage this was as much as he was able to tell them; they would have to accept that there was just not enough information to give them any further guide. It is important for families to realize that right from the beginning and for weeks to come, it will only be possible for the doctors to give them an uncertain guess about what the future holds. They can tell that an injury is severe or not so severe. They know that a certain percentage of people with severe injuries are likely to die, that some will recover with a handicap, and that others will do well. Saying that one particular patient, your Jonas, will do this or that can only be a guess guided by these probabilities. It is natural that families desperately want to know what is going to happen. The hard news is that the family must wait and see.

Jonas's parents asked if they might see their son. They felt that it was good for them to be with him for a moment, even when he was deeply unconscious, surrounded by tubes, machines, and a team working flat out. Some people would find this distressing and prefer to stay away; there should be no guilt in this.

After his parents had seen Jonas, he was taken to the X-ray department for the CT scan. When it was known that an operation was needed, the neurosurgeon talked to the parents to tell them what the situation was and what he thought was needed.

When Jonas was first brought into hospital the situation was critical. Every moment counted, and there was no time to find the family, to tell them what ought to be done and to get permission to do it. Treatment had to go ahead in good faith. There is now not quite so much urgency, and before operating on Jonas there is a little time for discussion with the family and to ask for their consent. The situation and risks need to be explained, both those of going ahead and those of doing nothing. However fully and sympathetically the situation is explained, the family may feel they have little say in the matter. As the decisions are forced on the team by the nature of the injury there is probably no way round this, but the staff should be fully open about the situation and answer questions patiently. The family are entitled to expect this. They should also try to realize that although the staff are professionals meeting similar situations every day, they still become emotionally involved, and need support and recognition if they are to do their job well.

Staff need to explain the situation:
as soon as possible
in as much detail as possible
as often as asked

Families need to realize:
there are no certainties, only probabilities
professionals are human

Surgery

Brain operations are unfamiliar and the thought of them often distresses people. In fact the operations needed for head injuries are usually straightforward and in themselves involve little risk. The real cause for anxiety is the condition which made them necessary and how much damage it has already done. This will usually only become plain much later on, when consciousness has returned and it can be seen how the brain is functioning. In Jonas's case the blood clot which was pressing on the brain was removed by cutting a trapdoor in the bone of the skull over the clot (the CT had shown the exact place) and then by washing the clot away. The bone, which was put back and fastened in place, had healed firmly by three or four weeks and left no weakness. The wounds he had sustained on the scalp and face were cleaned and closed, with the help of a plastic surgeon. Wounds like this can sometimes extend deeply, break through the bone and involve the brain itself, a 'compound depressed fracture'. These can look very frightening, especially if brain is showing in them. Sometimes there has been only a short period of unconsciousness and the patient is relatively intact, and in this case they can usually be dealt with successfully with little long-term disability. Fortunately in Jonas's case the wounds involved the skin only and had not extended through the bone.

Intensive care

Whether an operation is needed or not, people with severe head injuries will need to be looked after for a time in Intensive Care. Their whole system has been upset. As well as the head, other parts of the body have been damaged by the accident itself and by the low blood pressure and lack of oxygen that so often follows, and their whole body system is upset. The changes in the condition of the patient have to be watched very carefully and treatment needs to be adjusted from hour to hour. The assisted breathing that was started in the Accident Department is an important part of this programme of care, and it will need to be continued for several days, so that the brain has the best chance of recovering.

Intensive care monitoring

In order to keep a check on all these factors Jonas has to be connected with tubes and wires to several machines, each recording on a computer screen. The action of the heart shows continually on the electrocardiogram. With it the blood pressure is recorded, taken by putting a fine tube into a small artery in his ankle or arm. Often the pressure inside the head, the 'intracranial pressure', is measured continuously with a lead from inside the skull, and shown on the same screen. To feed Jonas and give him the medication he needs, a drip transfusion is put into a vein in his arm. Lastly there are the controls of the ventilator, the number of breaths a minute and how deep they are, which have to be managed to keep the amount of oxygen and carbon dioxide in the blood at the correct levels. There will be other tests as well. CT scans will be repeated to check on the amount of brain swelling and to make sure that no further blood clots have developed.

EEG

Tests of the electrical function of the brain are sometimes used. In the electroencephalogram (EEG) small electric currents arising in the brain are picked up by wires attached to the scalp and recorded on paper. This can help to tell how the brain is working and if function is returning.

SEPs

Another test is measurement of the 'Sensory Evoked Potentials' (SEPs). If a nerve in the arm or the leg is stimulated by a small electric current, there will be an alteration in the EEG. The time it takes for the change to occur is increased when the deep parts of the brain (the 'brain stem') are damaged. The first results will give an idea of how bad the damage is, and repeated tests will show how recovery is taking place.

EEGs and SEPs are useful in expert hands but are not essential to good care, and may only be available in larger hospitals.

These methods of looking after people who have been severely injured have only developed in the last 25 years or so, and a new sort of medical specialist, the 'intensivist' that we mentioned before, has developed to manage them. This new approach to accident care has resulted in an enormous increase in the number of lives saved.

Mechanical ventilation

One of the difficult decisions that has to be made is how long to use the ventilator for. The quiet breathing, the prevention of coughing and straining, and making sure of the right amount of oxygen and carbon dioxide in the blood create the best conditions for healing the brain. The ventilator may also be needed to manage chest or other injuries. It does have its disadvantages, however, and the intensivists will want to stop using it as soon as it is safe to do so. When things seem to be settling they will weigh up the pros and cons, and if they think the conditions are right they will start to allow the patient to breathe normally and see if they can manage on their own. Sometimes it turns out to be too early, and ventilation has to be continued for another day or two until another attempt can be made to discontinue it.

If ventilation has to be continued for more than three or four days the tube may start to irritate the windpipe and perhaps damage it. It may then be best to put in a 'tracheostomy' tube. At a small operation, usually with a local anaesthetic, the windpipe is opened through an incision in the neck just below the 'Adams apple' and a plastic tube threaded in. The ventilator is then connected to this. When the ventilator is no longer needed the tube can be used for unassisted breathing for a while until it is certain that the airway is clear. The tube can then be slipped out, and after a few days the hole in the neck will heal by itself.

Fluids and feeding

The method of feeding changes as things improve. To begin with all the fluid and nourishment that Jonas needed had to be given by a drip feed into a vein. After a day or two, as his condition became more stable, a fine tube was passed down his throat into his stomach (a 'nasogastric tube'). Specially formulated liquid food that could supply all his needs was given through this.

Special nursing care

People who lie unconscious need special nursing care. Skin can be damaged if there is pressure on the same point for too long. Joints will get stiff if they are not moved regularly. Splints for limb fractures need adjusting. Nurses and physiotherapists will constantly attend to this.

To keep Jonas alive all these measures were needed. A day after the operation another CT was done, which showed that the brain had settled down well after the clot had been removed. It was not yet possible to tell how his brain was working because of the sedation and muscle relaxing drugs. However, he was not yet ready to breathe on his own and it was three more days before it was possible to discontinue the ventilator. He was still unconscious but he would move his arms and his legs if the skin was pinched and there did not seem to be any obvious paralysis.

In another couple of days Jonas began to open his eyes and to move around a little in his bed. He had not yet tried to swallow and feeding was continued through the nasogastric tube. His condition was stable, he no longer needed life support, and he was ready to pass on to the next stage.

Intensive care: around the clock
Monitoring heart, blood pressure, ICP
Controlling breathing
Controlling fluids and food
Testing brain function
Nursing care
Waiting for the patient to take over his own body
 management

Head-injury ward

At the next stage patients are taken to a Head-Injury Ward. Its name and where it fits into the rest of the hospital will vary from place to place. In large hospitals it may be the neurosurgical ward, in smaller ones a general surgical ward that will take all sorts of cases. It could be a special unit for head-injury care and rehabilitation, though these are not common yet. Who is in charge will vary, but in general there will be a senior doctor responsible for the overall medical care, and a charge nurse who runs the ward. There will be junior doctors, in the British system called registrars and house surgeons, in North America residents and interns, and nurses responsible to the charge nurse. There will also be people expert in other forms of treatment: physiotherapists who will look after joints, muscles and movements and the chest; occupational therapists who will help to restore the everyday activities of living; speech therapists, dietitian, and psychologists. All these people will come into contact with Jonas and play a part in his recovery.

One of the problems which Jonas's family will have is knowing who to go to for information, and to sort out what the advice from the various team members adds up to. Larger units, accustomed to dealing with the head-injured and their families, will have worked this out. Regular briefing sessions should be arranged so that the family knows exactly what is happening, and so that the members of the team can pass on their instructions directly. Family members will often be tempted to try to get information about progress outside these sessions, and to ask a nurse at the bedside or a junior doctor met casually in the corridor how things are going. The nurse or the doctor may want to help, but they may not have the up-to-date answers and they may say something which ends up in misunderstanding or chaos. It is much the wisest course to look for important information only from the person in charge, or someone specially nominated by them for the purpose.

Smaller units may not have the process as well organized as this. You are strongly recommended to insist on seeing the person ultimately responsible for care, and ask this person what you need to know. It should be possible to make a regular appointment for this.

Staff need to arrange regular communication:
as much information as possible should be given
as often as asked
by the same person each time if possible

Let us now go back to Jonas, who had reached the stage when he was responding to his family with simple words and moving around his bed on his own. He soon began to eat a little and it was safe to remove the nasogastric tube. It was important to make sure that he was swallowing properly and that food was not getting into his lungs; at this stage in some units X-ray tests are done to make sure the swallowing mechanism has recovered properly. The physiotherapists were helping him to get back his balance and strength, and the occupational therapists were teaching him to look after himself, to wash and to dress. He was encouraged to do anything that would help him to get his skills back — puzzles, hobbies, music or games. Though his arms seemed to be moving normally, at first his left hand was clumsy and he had difficulty using it. It was plain that though the blood clot had been removed the right side of his brain had not yet completely recovered. The occupational and physical therapists needed to work with him on this.

We mentioned before that the members of the team passed on their instructions to the family. These instructions, and carrying them out, become vital at this stage. There are never enough staff to give all the treatment that is needed, and the family will have to do a great deal to back up the treatment of the professionals. There are also things that only the family can do, such as reminding him of his life before the accident and re-introducing him to his old world. Family are entitled to ask about the reasons for each recommendation. Sometimes they may feel that it is not the right thing to do, and if this is the case they should talk it out with the staff. The family should never agree to one thing and do another; this can do untold harm to the patient, the one person who really matters.

A fortnight after going to the head-injury ward Jonas was up and walking around. He was not yet behaving normally and he had a number of problems with mental function which are described later in the book. As he was able to do more, he began to go on expeditions outside the hospital with his family, first for an hour or two, then overnight and eventually for weekends. He no longer needed the sort of care which is given in the acute ward of a hospital and he could now move on to the next stage of his recovery. This transition and the problems it raises are described in the next chapter.

The Head-Injury Ward
Returns the patient to:
independent feeding
independent moving
self-care
ability to communicate
his family

Failure to recover

In Chapter 2 we mentioned that some people with severe head injuries survive the immediate threat to life but then seem to make no further recovery. Investigations such as EEGs and further CT and perhaps an MR scan will be done to see if there is some remediable cause; often the conclusion will be that the initial damage was just too great. In spite of this, after a time, for some reason which is often not apparent, patients do occasionally suddenly start to improve. Full care with the hope of a change will therefore be continued for a long time.

Usually but not always they will no longer depend on mechanical ventilation, but because of a poor cough reflex they may not be able to deal with secretions and a tracheostomy may need to remain in place. The nasogastric tube often irritates the throat if it is used for a long time and a feeding tube may be placed directly in the stomach. This can be done through a small operation on the abdomen, or inserted using a gastroscope, a flexible telescope which is passed down the throat into the stomach. People in this state often have a spastic paralysis, in which the muscles are contracting strongly all the time and pull the joints into abnormal positions. This makes nursing care difficult at the time and leaves the patient with disabling joint contractures if they do improve. Splints may be able to hold the joints in a normal position, but sometimes the muscles are too strong. It may be useful to weaken them for several months so that the joints can recover, and this can be done simply with injections into the muscles.

Some patients in this state do seem to have a degree of awareness of what goes on around them. They may respond by a change in muscle tension or breathing, or by eye movement. Even though it seems unlikely, it is best always to assume that they can understand something of what is going on, and to talk to them about simple things; they may seem to respond to things that they liked before the accident, such as music. It is important never to let them know that you have given up hope. You yourself should be realistic about the small chance of improvement, but remember that just occasionally people do return to better function after months or even years of being in this state.

After a time there will be pressure to have the long-stay patient moved out of an acute treatment area. In some places there are special provisions, but in many this will mean transfer to an area where there is less active care. It will be important to make sure that all the measures such as gastrostomy and control of spastic muscles are done before this move is made, and that there are arrangements for regular review by the specialist team.

Failure to recover
Special treatment:
  Gastrostomy
  Spastic muscles
Familiar things
Realism and hope

Moderately severe head injuries

Many people have head injuries which need managing in hospital, but their condition is not bad enough for them to need the full regime of treatment we have just described. Usually the person will have been seen in the accident department of the hospital and from there admitted either for a short period to Intensive Care or directly to the 'Head-Injury Ward' that we described. They may already be awake when they get to the ward or be semi-conscious and remain like that for a day or two. Their progress will be much like Jonas's but faster, and they will need help from the same therapy team.

There are two main considerations while they are in hospital. The first is that after even quite mild injuries complications can occur — the 'third injury' that we described before. These have to be recognized and treated at once. A large part of the care therefore will consist of regular observations and further tests such as CT scans if there is any concern.

In the early stages some of the patients will need the same sort of care that was given to the severely injured cases. They will need nursing care for observations, feeding, and toileting. They may become restless, confused, and aggressive, requiring special management. Later there may be problems with movement and balance, thinking and behaviour, and they will need help from the physiotherapists, occupational and speech therapists and psychologists.

The hospital staff that the family will need to deal with have been described above, and there should be the same care in making sure that the family gets reliable information.

It is important that before discharge from hospital patients of this group should have a definite plan for rehabilitation, worked out by the medical team and therapists. For some a check-up after a week or two will be sufficient, for others a more extensive outpatient program will be needed. Even the person who seems to recover quickly may later find that they have persisting problems. Managing these is discussed in Chapter 5.

Less severe injuries:
Recover more quickly but:
they have the same risks in the early stages
they need the same precautions
they may still have problems with thinking and behaviour when
   recovery otherwise seems complete

Mild head injuries

For every person who is admitted to hospital after a head injury three or more will be seen in the accident department and then allowed to go home. Many will have recovered completely by the time they get to hospital and have come just to be checked. Some will have been semi-conscious or confused when they arrive but return to normal after an hour or two. Some will need cuts on their scalp cleaned and stitched, or have minor injuries elsewhere.

The importance of the hospital visit for these people, apart from the care of cuts and minor injuries, is to deal with the risk of a 'third injury', for this complication can follow even minor head injury. Because of the seriousness of the risk hospitals have strict rules to sort out those who can safely be allowed to go home. They will vary a little from place to place, but the rules are generally along these lines:

1. People who are safe to go home must be free from any sign of complication, thinking clearly with normal memory, with good balance and only minor headache.
2. There must not be any sign of a skull fracture. The fracture itself does not matter, but complications are perhaps 30 times more common in those who have one. Some hospitals make it a rule to X-ray everyone for a fracture, but probably this is unnecessary and wasteful, and X-rays need only be done if there is a definite indication that a fracture might be present.
3. In some hospitals CT scans are done if there is any doubt whether a patient is fit to go home. However, patients with disabling symptoms which need continuing care may still have normal scans.
4. There must be a competent person at home to look after them.

Many hospitals have special rules for children and old people, who may have a particular risk of complications.

Remember!
You have a right to competent and compassionate treatment
  and choice
You have a right to information
The person you ask can only give you probabilities
Head injuries take a long time to heal

4

Leaving hospital — what happens now?

After the first dreadful days or weeks when you did not know whether your friend or relative was going to live or die, all you wanted was to have him well enough to leave hospital and come home. During that time you spent every waking minute that you could at his bedside, even at first when he was still unconscious, and it was important both for him and for you that you were able to do this. However, it had been a pace that no-one could keep up for long. The strain of perhaps rushing home from work, rustling up a quick meal, maybe getting children to bed or finding a babysitter, the long drive to the hospital and the struggle to find a car park, were beginning to take their toll, and you thought it would all be so much easier when he was home again. But now that the time has come for him to leave hospital you realize that it may not be as simple as you thought, you wonder if it is right for him, and whether or not you will be able to cope. Firstly we need to look at the reasons for the move from hospital and how it works, and secondly, at possible alternatives.

Why is it time to leave hospital?

You read in Chapter 3 how Jonas progressed from the Intensive Care Department to the Head-Injury Ward while he was in hospital. This move was made when there was no longer any need for the life-support machinery, although he still needed to have expert nursing care for the whole 24-hour day. As he improved he was able to do more and more for himself, and at last he had reached the stage where his only needs were a bed and a roof over his head, food, and a little help with the difficult things. Not only were the services of an acute hospital ward not needed any longer, but the atmosphere of sickness and the absence of peace and quiet were not good for him. He was ready to move on. It is important to remember, though, that just because he has been discharged from hospital it does not mean that he has recovered from the head injury. The important work has just begun.

Where to go: home or somewhere else?

As well as the basics of living, the head-injured person has two other needs. One is to get back to living in the world outside hospital, supported by family and friends and with the sense of security that this brings. Most parents will want to provide this support, because this is what they have done over the years when their children were growing up, through the trials of chicken pox and mumps, broken bones, school reports, and adolescence. Wives will want to look after the husbands whom they love, and vice versa. Friends will want to show that nothing has changed.

Going back home is usually the first choice. It is the nearest thing to normal, the surroundings are familiar, and the patient will be among family. Sometimes, of course, this is not possible because of circumstances; there may not be room, a parent or spouse may be ill, or there may be some other barrier.

Although home may be the obvious choice, in some circumstances it is not always the best choice. Indeed there can be real disadvantages. The first is that a person who has had a head injury can be very difficult to deal with. Often he is not aware of how he is behaving, and he can lose the consideration for others which makes family life possible. He is often irritable and sensitive to noise made by other people. He may want to do unsuitable or unsafe things, like playing the stereo very loudly in the middle of the night, or insisting on taking his motor bike out for a spin, (you will read more about these problems in the next chapter). In many cases he has been used to living his own life, making his own decisions, and it can be very difficult for family to exert enough firmness to control this sort of situation. The shift from the role of loving parent or spouse to that of a firm guardian is a very difficult one to make, and a situation can develop that is destructive both to the family and to the head-injured person.

In-hospital needs	After-hospital needs
Life support	Food and shelter
Intensive care	Supervision
24-hour nursing	Family and friends
	Rehabilitation

We have already said that there are two needs, one being to return to living in the everyday world. The other is for formal rehabilitation treatment, the treatment that will get movement and balance back to normal, which will help the patient with his thinking, and which will help him return to the occupation and skills which he had before the accident. Some of this can be achieved by a home programme arranged by the hospital therapists but much of it needs to be done under expert supervision. This often means frequent visits to the hospital or rehabilitation centre. If it is a long way away there may be problems with transport, and the travelling can make the person so tired that the treatment does less good. If this is the case then it may be best to live at a rehabilitation centre. Going home for weekends can then become a real holiday and enjoyed by everyone.

In ideal circumstances the pros and cons of leaving hospital and going either home or to a residential rehabilitation centre would be worked out on the facts of each case, and a trial made of what seemed the better choice, always with the chance of changing if it seemed good to do so. It is unfortunate that this rational choice is often not possible. There may be no centre, or a waiting list which is often so long that there is a destructive gap between application and acceptance. Out-patient rehabilitation may be all that is available.

People with less severe head injuries

Many people will stay in the Head-Injury Ward for only a few days and they will recover to the extent that home is the obvious place to go. This does not mean that some of the problems we have described above will not occur. A person who seems to have made a very good recovery in the controlled surroundings of a hospital ward may still become irritable when he has to deal with noisy children or neighbours, and he may not accept that he is neither fit to drive nor well enough to go to the pub for a drink. In most cases this stage lasts for a short time only, and provided that you have been warned about the problems and advised how to cope (see Chapter 5) you should get by without too much trouble.

Many hospitals have a system where the patient is given an appointment to come back to see the doctor in two or three weeks' time. At this stage usually some tests will be done to check the person's ability to concentrate, and to check how well memory and reaction times have recovered. This is the stage when the decision will be made about whether he should begin the return to work or school, or be started on a rehabilitation programme.

A person with a less severe injury, who has not been admitted to hospital, misses out on this care. Because of the numbers involved, it would be very expensive to include every patient in the system outlined in the last paragraph. However, it should be possible to provide a service for the 5–10 per cent of patients from this group who may miss out on this care. (One such service is described in Chapter 7).

People who are not well enough to go home

As we have already pointed out in Chapter 3, some people with very severe head injuries make little progress after they leave intensive care. They move and speak very little, they do not respond very much to what is going on around them, and they remain dependent on others even for basic needs such as feeding or toileting. Their care in the Head-Injury Ward, where people are expected to be progressing, becomes inappropriate and the hospital needs to move them somewhere else.

Because of the burden of their care, only very rarely, for example in the case of very young children, is it possible for the patient to go home. Some health districts have special accommodation for the patient, but in many cases publicly funded or private geriatric hospitals are the only possibilities. These may (sometimes they do not) provide a level of care that is adequate to keep them alive and free from complications. However, it is rare for them to continue with a programme that is based on the expectation of further improvement. It is a fact, however, that if a patient does receive continued rehabilitation then he can continue to improve, although very slowly, and he sometimes may achieve sufficient recovery to make the difference between total dependence and at least partial self-care.

How is leaving the hospital organized?

When your relative or friend is ready to leave hospital he may be transferred to a rehabilitation centre, or be looked after at home. If he is to go to a rehabilitation facility or to another hospital, the date and the time is set to suit both places. But you as the parent or family member are entitled to be kept fully informed of the plans. Even though the transfer is to another medical facility, you should make sure that you work through the rest of this chapter which suggests the things that should be done before a patient leaves the hospital which he has been in since the accident.

If you are going to look after your friend or relative at home, there need to be arrangements which will make sure that you will be able to cope before he is handed over to your care. A system which works well, and which is followed by many acute-care hospitals, has three stages. The time of each stage should be set by a meeting of family members, medical and nursing staff, rehabilitation therapists, and usually the social worker assigned to your case. The patient may also be present if he is able to take part in the discussion. Before the first meeting or 'case conference' the occupational therapist may have visited your home to see what modifications will be needed to make it practical for the head-injured person to live with you. If he will still be in a wheelchair when he goes home, for example, then access to the house must be looked at and modifications made so that he can use the bathroom and the toilet.

The first home-stay stage is usually a day visit. You might pick him up in your car, or ambulance transport might be arranged to bring him home and later return him to the hospital. If you manage this without too many problems, then the patient can have weekend leave, where he stays at home overnight on a Saturday evening. Again after discussion of any problems, and after modifications have been made to overcome these problems, you move on to the final stage, which is full discharge home from hospital.

The three stages to going home from hospital
Day visit
Weekend leave
Discharge

Before he leaves hospital, make an appointment to see the doctor who is in charge of your friend or relative. Make a list of the things you want to know about. Remember that this specialist is a busy person who is likely to have unscheduled emergencies which interrupt your visit with him, so allow enough time before the date set for discharge to fit in another appointment if necessary.

You will want to ask the specialist about the medication which the patient may be taking, and who you should go to to renew the prescription, or to make a decision about when it can be stopped. You will also want to ask about a follow-up appointment for him to be seen by the doctor in charge, or by a member of the team. If he is to go to a rehabilitation centre, find out how you can get to see and talk to who-ever will be looking after him there.

If you will be looking after your friend or relative at home you will need to check that arrangements have been made for him to have any out-patient treatment which may be needed, and that you know the name and contact phone number of the person who has overall responsibility for his rehabilitation.

Many areas have support groups for families and care-givers where you can talk with other people who have had the same experiences as you (see Appendix B). If you have not already done so, make sure that you make contact with your local group before the patient leaves hos-pital. This is the time when you will need all the support that you can get. It is also important to make sure that arrangements are made before the patient comes home from hospital for the practical help which you might need. In some countries, for example, if he still has difficulty with bladder control then you can get bedding and sleepwear provided and laundered by the extramural hospital. Ask the social worker about what help may be available in your case.

The time that the head-injured person is in hospital is the time when you should have most direct access to rehabilitation officers and to social workers. Make sure that these people understand your family circumstances. This is the time to find out what financial help you are entitled to. For example, if you will need to take time off work to look after your friend or family member some accident insurance schemes allow for you to be reimbursed for loss of wages. Your social worker will be able to tell you about other allowances. Do not be too proud to take advantage of these. Money will not compensate you for the effects of the accident but it may make the difference between being able to afford labour-saving help and struggling to balance the budget on a reduced income, with the extra expense that is entailed in caring for someone who has had a head injury.

If the friend or relative that you will be looking after at home is still not able to walk, make sure that you have been shown how to get him and the wheelchair into your car. If you do not have your own trans-port, check that arrangements have been made by the hospital to bring him back for out-patient appointments. Check also about how this is to be paid for. The expense of even a short journey can become a burden if this journey has to be repeated five or six days a week for months on end. Again, check with your social worker or rehabilitation officer to see if you can be reimbursed for travel.

> **Before you take the patient home from hospital**
> *Have you:*
> asked about medication?
> asked about out-patient treatment?
> been given the name of your contact person?
> contacted a family support group?
> found out about financial help?
> found out about practical help?

Rehabilitation

To most families rehabilitation is a magic word. If only their relative or friend could get to a rehabilitation centre, or have physiotherapy every day, or start speech therapy, then their problems would all be solved. It is tempting but unrealistic to blame a shortfall in rehabilitation resources rather than the head injury for the condition. This is not to say that rehabilitation is not important, but it is equally important to be aware of what is possible, and what traumatic brain damage means.

When brain cells are destroyed in an accident they do not grow again. This is not nearly as bad as it seems, because most of us have millions more brain cells than we can use, and one of the theories about why people do get some recovery after brain injury is that new brain pathways can be set up using these 'spare' cells. These new pathways will be established only if the person continuously practises the actions that have been disrupted. Thus repetition and more repetition is the basis of most physical rehabilitation techniques.

However, repetition is not the answer when we are working on rehabilitation of cognitive functions like memory and reasoning and attention. Memory is not a muscle, and all constant repetition is likely to do is frustrate the head-injured person and increase his anxiety level, and make him too tired to cope with the rest of his programme.

The rehabilitation team

Depending on the injuries of your friend or family member he will work with some or all of the following rehabilitation team members:

Physiotherapists (physical therapists)

The physiotherapist aims to help patients recover the ability to use the muscles in their arms, legs, neck, and trunk, so that they can sit and stand without losing their balance, and co-ordinate their movements. Exercises may range from practice in leg movements, so that they can walk again, to practice in fine hand movements, so that they can use a pen.

Occupational therapists

The occupational therapist aims to help patients carry out everyday tasks. Exercises can range from showing them how to dress themselves and to carry out their own toilet, to teaching them about budgeting and managing their own finances. The occupational therapist will also provide special equipment to help them to be as independent as possible, even though they may have considerable physical handicaps.

Speech therapists

The speech and language therapist aims to help patients communicate with other people, using both spoken and written words. This means that they could have exercises in reading and writing, as well as exercises aimed at giving them practice in understanding what people are saying to them. The speech therapist may also give them practice in remembering what they have read and heard.

Neuropsychologists

The neuropsychologist has a special interest in cognitive skills; those skills such as memory, perception, and understanding that are needed for us to gain knowledge. He or she aims to find what abilities the patient has, what skills have been affected by the injury, and in what way. If there is a memory problem, for example, is this just a problem when words have to be remembered, is the problem mainly in getting things into memory, or in getting things out again at some later stage? The aim is to find out what areas need working on. The neuropsychologist will see the patients regularly during rehabilitation to check that the programme they are on is helping them with any cognitive problems that they have.

Cognitive retraining therapists

In some centres cognitive retraining is carried out by the neuropsychologist, in some by the occupational therapist, and in other areas the speech therapist does this. In each case the aim is to teach the patient how to compensate for the skills that have been lost or impaired. Sometimes this is done by teaching them to use the skills that have not been affected by the accident to help them carry out activities that are hard for them because of the brain injury. Sometimes it is done by modifying the environment in which they live, for example, installing time switches on electrical appliances so that an alarm will sound if they are not turned off in time. There are now also excellent electronic notebooks to use as memory minders.

Social workers

Social workers are skilled in helping families get the practical help that is needed. They know which community and government facilities are available, and they will often be involved in finding somewhere for the patient to go when it is time to leave hospital. Social workers are also often involved in running support groups, either for the head-injured persons themselves or for their families.

Clinical psychologists

The clinical psychologist is a skilled counsellor, and will help both the patient and the family cope with the changes that the accident has brought about. He or she will also be able to help if the patient's behaviour is causing management problems.

Rehabilitation officers

Some accident insurance schemes employ rehabilitation officers who will act as co-ordinators of different services. Their involvement will sometimes continue until the head-injured person has made a full recovery, or until the recovery has 'plateaued', that is, until there has been no improvement over several months.

The rehabilitation team
Physiotherapist (physical therapist)
Occupational therapist
Speech therapist
Neuropsychologist
Cognitive retraining therapist
Social worker
Clinical psychologist
Rehabilitation officer

What can you expect from rehabilitation?

Rehabilitation aims to help people who have had head injuries reach their potential level of recovery. At one end of the scale are people who eventually will be able to do all the activities which they did before their accidents at a similar level of skill. At the other end of the scale there will be people who may be able to do nothing except breathe for themselves, even years after the injury. For these people, extensive expenditure of rehabilitation time and effort is needed to make any difference to how they do, and their potential for recovery is limited.

In most cases there is the problem that 'potential level of recovery' is difficult to measure. We can of course keep a record of 'partial recovery', how much recovery people have made at fixed periods of time after the injury. Does failure to find any improvement from one period to the next mean that the patients have reached their potential? Is this as well as they are likely to get? Not necessarily. It does suggest, however, that the patients have reached the stage when the effort that is being spent on their rehabilitation is not accompanied by returns that justify the effort.

At this point the rehabilitation team will probably suggest that the treatment is cut back, or they may give your relative or friend a three or six month break from treatment. They may explain to you that they need to concentrate their efforts on patients who will get more benefit from the time that is spent with them. This is often a difficult decision for families to accept. It is important to remember that the pattern of recovery after neurological damage is usually one of rapid gains early after injury, and much slower gains, and even pauses, in recovery after that. It is important that you make sure that you have been given a definite appointment time when progress can be checked, and when the decision to reduce treatment can be reviewed.

Rehabilitation — magic cures

It is often at the stage when recovery seems to have stopped that the search for a magic cure begins. There is the belief that somehow, somewhere, there will be rehabilitation for your family member or friend's head injury that will fix things. Usually this magic cure is in another country or state. Often it is something that you will have read about in the popular press. It usually involves considerable expense because it is not recognized as part of orthodox rehabilitation medicine, and so is not covered by your accident insurance. Often it involves considerable sacrifices of personal and family life, because you and your family have to be the practitioners of this therapy. One of the inevitable consequences of this is that you are then responsible for the success or failure of the treatment. It is natural that families feel some guilt about the circumstances of the accident, no matter how tenuous the cause for blame. It is tragic when another source of guilt is added if the magic does not work.

Of course, just because a treatment is unorthodox or costly or time-consuming does not necessarily make it useless or ineffective. By the same token, it does not necessarily mean that it does work. Before you commit yourself to any new course of action, first of all talk it over with the co-ordinator of the rehabilitation programme. Find out what the magic cure offers that the conventional programme does not. It may be possible to try out new exercises at home with the help of rehabilitation staff your family member or friend is familiar with, without the effort and expense of travelling miles to a strange place. Sometimes the only difference is in the quantity of treatment, and more is not necessarily better for the head-injured person. Remember that one of his main problems is that he tires very quickly, and when the brain is tired the only thing that extra exercise will do is to tire him even further.

It is also helpful to discuss the decision to try out the new treatment with your family doctor, who should also be able to warn you if it may prove harmful in your case. You need also to bring it up with your family support group so that you can find out if there are other families who have tried the magic cure. Finally, never commit yourself to a programme or centre on the spur of the moment. Wait till you have all the information that you can get, and take all the advice that you can, particularly advice from people who do not have anything to gain from your decision, or who do not have a special interest in the proposed treatment.

Rehabilitation in isolated country areas

We have talked about the lack of appropriate rehabilitation centres, and pointed out that this is a problem which is universal. The problem is even greater if you live in an area away from a main centre, as even the most ambitious and wealthy health system cannot be expected to provide facilities in every town and village in the country. What do you do if you live in a geographically isolated area?

The first decision that you will be faced with is, should you move to a bigger centre where your friend or relative can get the help that is needed? Obviously this will depend on your family circumstances, but in general you should not be hasty in doing this. Certainly you need to discuss the move with all the members of your family. The head-injured person is not the only one who needs to be considered. You also need to discuss alternative plans with your social worker. It may be possible to find residential accommodation for the patient, or for him to be given a rehabilitation programme that he can do at home.

If you follow a rehabilitation programme at home then your first need will be for information and advice. One of the reasons for writing this book was to cater for people who do not have access to face-to-face counselling about head injury. But since no book can be a substitute for interaction with other people, it is important that you arrange for some sort of personal contact. This may be with a staff member of the hospital where your relative or friend was nursed immediately after the accident. Some rehabilitation teams have community workers who will visit people in isolated areas at intervals of once a month or so, and you should get to know them before they leave hospital. It is also important that you attend at least one support group meeting before the discharge date, so that you can set up a network of people you can write to when you need to get things off your chest. Finally, it is especially important to make sure that the social worker finds out about what extra help you may be entitled to as a resident in an isolated area.

Case histories

Samuel

Samuel's next-door neighbour, Mr Smith, was working in his front garden when he heard a yell and looked up to see Samuel flying across the road, and then saw him land in a crumpled heap on the opposite footpath. Mr Smith vaulted his front gate and rushed across to find Samuel lying unconscious, and with his leg twisted in an ominous way. Other neighbours called the ambulance while Mr Smith supported Samuel's head and carefully turned his face to one side. In a few minutes Samuel started moaning, and by the time the ambulance arrived was awake and crying with pain. His parents were still not home, and Mr Smith went off in the ambulance with him.

By the time his parents reached the hospital Samuel had had pain-relief, his leg had been X-rayed, and he was being wheeled back into the cubicle in the Emergency Ward while arrangements were made to admit him to an orthopaedic ward. Neither his parents nor the hospital staff were aware that Samuel had also had a head injury, as the ambulance report noted him to be conscious and in pain' when they reached him. Mr Smith had been so concerned by the lad's pain and distress that he had not thought to tell the ambulance officers about the period of coma.

Samuel had emergency surgery on his fractured femur, and a pin was inserted to stabilize it. His mother was relieved to find that this meant that he would not need to have it in plaster, but also worried about how she would keep her daredevil son from using it before he should. She was also embarrassed because Samuel was not a good patient. He was weepy and irritable, and screamed whenever anyone except his parents came near him. They thought he was delirious because he kept asking where he was, and why they hadn't come to see him before. However, after the first couple of days he was more manageable, and the physiotherapist began teaching him to use crutches. He kept forgetting that he was not supposed to put any weight on his leg, and someone needed to be at his side whenever he was out of bed to make sure he was safe. He spent most of the time asleep, which was put down to the rather unusually large amount of pain-relief that he needed.

Fortunately Samuel settled down by the end of the week, and was able to go home with his crutches, with his parents laden down with the goodies his neighbours and friends had given him in hospital. His mother took time off work to stay at home to care for him, and he was shifted into a downstairs bedroom so he would not have to cope with the stairs. They continued to be rather puzzled by his behaviour, however. For example, when he saw his rather battered roller blades he was furious that someone had been using *his* birthday present while he was in hospital, and insisted that he had not ever had a chance to try them out. His parents thought that the shock of breaking his leg must have led him to repress the accident and how it happened. He was also rather weepy and demanding, and after two weeks at home his parents were relieved when his orthopaedic surgeon cleared him to return to school. They were sure he was getting 'spoilt' by the attention of being a patient, and even his long suffering older brothers had had enough of being ordered to turn off the stereo because the noise gave Samuel a headache.

Jonas

The team at the acute hospital were concerned that Jonas's parents would find him difficult to control, and because he was able to get around on his own there was a likelihood that he would get himself into situations where he could be at risk. Fortunately he lived in a city which had a good residential rehabilitation unit, so instead of going directly to his home he was transferred there from the acute hospital. His parents were pleased because it was close to where they lived which made it easier for them to visit. They were also pleased to learn how well staffed it was, and to find there was a specialized wing for people who had had brain injury. However, both they and Jonas were rather shocked to find that many of the other residents had obviously been in very severe accidents. Only a few were able to walk on their own, and many could not talk clearly.

Jonas made a fuss at first and said that he was not going to stay, but then he discovered that a rather attractive young lady called Suzy was something called his 'primary worker'. Suzy explained that her job was to make sure everything was going smoothly, and that he should talk to her if he was worried about things. She also told him that he would not need to stay in the unit for very long, but that the staff needed to find out what he could do for himself, and what help he should have, so that they could make sure he had the rehabilitation programme that would be best for him. The first week passed quite quickly, with the days filled with assessments with the occupational, speech and physical therapists and with the neuropsychologist. These made him quite tired, and he was often found asleep in his bedroom rather than at the therapy session he was scheduled to attend. However, the staff were all experienced and well trained, and left him be, as they knew that attempting to give him rehabilitation exercises would be pointless if he was tired.

There was a case conference at the beginning of the second week, with Jonas, his parents, the rehabilitation doctor and the social worker, as well as Suzy and the therapists who had worked with him. After some ten minutes or so of listening to reports of what they had found, Jonas's attention started to wander. However, he pricked up his ears when he heard Suzy say that she thought he was ready to move on to an out-patient programme, but that he should not go back to his flat. Instead he would need to stay with his parents for a while. The neuropsychologist and occupational therapist both agreed with Suzy, and Jonas became very angry, both because his objection was outnumbered, and because Suzy was siding with the others. The case conference ended after he stormed out, and it was decided to leave things as they were for another week.

Eventually a bargain was struck. Jonas agreed that he would stay with his parents until he had learned to prepare his own meals, and to dress himself on his own. Even he had to admit that he needed help getting dressed, even when he was just trying to put on a track-suit. He insisted that he could make his own meals, but agreed to have some supervised meal preparation sessions with the occupational therapist in return for her helping to sort out how he could put his clothes on without having to ask for help. The social worker had arranged with the accident insurer for them to provide some additional attendant care; a young man of the same age as Jonas who would take him to his out-patient sessions. This made him feel better about the bargain. He did not want the other patients, and especially he did not want Suzy, to think that he had to have his parents take him to places.

Pauline

One minute Pauline had been hurrying along the street; the next thing she knew she was lying on a stretcher which was being wheeled into the Emergency Department. There was an oxygen mask over her face, and she struggled to remove it as it felt uncomfortable and smothering. Then she remembered the court case. She panicked when she was told the time, which was some half an hour after the case was due to begin. However, she was persuaded to stay where she was at least until she had been examined when she was promised that messages would be sent to her firm, and that her husband would be told about the accident. She had torches shone in her eyes, her blood pressure and temperature checked, and was asked continual silly questions, such as what day it was, and where she was. She remembered being a bit unclear about the day at first, and was not sure which hospital she was in. The previous week she had taken her teenage son to a local emergency clinic when he had sprained his ankle, and for some time she was sure that must be where she was.

She also felt rather nauseated, and became quite distressed when she was unable to get to the vomit bowl in time and was sick on the bed. In spite of the nurse comforting her and getting her into a clean hospital gown, she was emotional and weepy. When her husband John walked in she burst into tears. To him this was the most worrying aspect of the afternoon, as Pauline had always been a very 'together' person. He sat by her side until he saw a doctor passing the cubicle, and he managed to speak to him before he could move on to another patient. The doctor assured him that Pauline had only been concussed, and that if her recordings were stable after four hours she would be able to go home.

The four hours passed eventually. Pauline slept most of the time between the nurse's visits, and by the third hour managed to get all the silly questions right. By this time also she was visited by a colleague from her law firm who had been working with her on the case. He reassured her that all was well, and that the case had been put off until the next morning, and that he would be able to handle it.

It was closer to six hours than four hours before Pauline was eventually helped into her husband's car for the ride home. They had been given some printed leaflets about what to do and some pages of information about what to expect in the next day or two, but Pauline was more interested in getting home to her own bed. She had a splitting headache by this time, and just wanted a chance to sleep it off without being woken up by the light of a torch in her eyes!

5 The continuing effects of head injury

When the staff at the hospital talked to you about what the future might hold for your relative or friend they probably used the terms 'brain damage' or 'brain injury'. Obviously the outcome depends on the amount of damage but the words suggest a gloomy outlook to most people. The amount of recovery that you have seen up until the time the head-injured person is ready to leave hospital will have been a great source of reassurance to you, and you are right to assume that it will continue. You need to realize, however, that although the patient is well enough to leave hospital, there are many problems still to be faced. If you know about these in advance then you will be better prepared to deal with them.

In this chapter we describe the problems ahead and explain why they occur. We also give you some suggestions about how to cope with them. These are problems which almost every person who has had a head injury will experience, although the severity will vary and each will have an individual mixture. In Chapter 6 we will describe the special problems which only a proportion of people will experience.

Fatigue

Without doubt, fatigue is one of the most limiting after-effects of head injury because it influences everything that is done. The person will find that after every activity he will tire much more quickly than he expects, whether he is trying to concentrate, take exercise, or just talk socially. Even activities which are normally relaxing, such as watching television, can tire him. Why this should be is not yet known but it seems likely that the injury has damaged that part of the brain which controls the rhythm of sleeping and waking. This is not surprising as the first effect of a head injury is coma, a very deep sort of sleep.

Someone who is fit and well wakes in the morning feeling fresh. He can work right through the day until he starts to feel tired, a word we use to describe the feeling that everything needs much more effort. If a person goes on working when he is tired he gets careless, and the quality of the work deteriorates. At last it becomes too unpleasant, there are too many mistakes however hard he tries, and he has to stop. After a good night's rest he is fresh again and can get back to work. It looks as if he starts the day with a measured amount of energy, he can work until this is exhausted, when this happens he becomes tired and inefficient, and then he can get the energy back by a good night's sleep.

A head-injured person can feel reasonably fresh when he wakes, but within a short time, an hour or two or maybe less, the feeling of tiredness comes on and, much more quickly than the well person, his performance deteriorates and he has to stop. When he takes a sleep or rest it does him less good than he expects. Even if he gets a good night's sleep he may not feel fresh the next morning. What seems to be happening is that he starts with much less energy, uses it up more quickly, and has difficulty getting it back by resting. The next day he is still in 'energy-debt' so that the symptoms start even sooner.

There are other disturbances of the sleeping or waking mechanism. After head injury more time may be spent in the lighter stages of sleep, which are less refreshing. As a result of this the quality of dreaming may change, sometimes with nightmares, and sometimes with very little dreaming at all.

> If your head-injured friend says that he is too tired to go out with you, he probably is.

It is often very difficult for a person who has had a head injury to understand the needs of this situation. We are all brought up to believe that we can 'do better if we try harder' and the reaction to fatigue is often dogged perseverance and a determination to finish the job. This usually results in a downward spiral of deterioration.

Families and rehabilitation staff need to act as monitors of the head-injured person's energy use, to make sure that he stays within the limits where he will be able to function effectively. The rehabilitation team will organize the treatment times so that periods which are 'energy-draining' are alternated with periods of rest, when his batteries can be recharged. Families will monitor the home and leisure activities to make sure that he is not overdoing things. To do this, families need to appreciate that the signs that he is over-tired are not necessarily that he will want to lie down or sit in a chair. Indeed, often the opposite is true. He can become more restless, more distractable, more disorganized, or more talkative. His mood may seem exaggerated, he may be quicker to laugh or to argue and less easy to reason with, or he may withdraw and refuse to discuss anything; yet he may deny that he is tired, even though this is very obvious to you.

It will be difficult to persuade him to do the only sensible thing, that is, to take some rest. This is why it is important that the care-givers monitor the amount of activity, and are able to direct the head-injured person to rest before he gets to the 'over-tired' stage. Often there are very clear signals that your relative or friend has exceeded the energy level and is approaching this overload. You need to watch out for these signals. Some of the most frequent are increasing irritability, unusual pallor, a drawn tense look, or a rather glazed expression in the eyes.

If you can recognize the early signs of fatigue in your relative or friend, you can help him by directing him to stop or change what he is doing, and to husband his energies. This should be the first priority in managing the problem. The second problem is to protect him from well meaning associates who do not understand the basis of his tiredness. As an example, if you know that he does not have the energy to watch a video (which involves concentrating on the screen, remembering the plot, the characters, what they said, and so on) you can dissuade his associates from pressuring him to join them. The third priority of fatigue management is that of communication. You need to keep the rehabilitation team informed of any unusually tiring activity that your relative or friend has taken up, or anything different that he has done which has made him more tired than normal, or importantly, has affected his ability to cope with rehabilitation.

Unfortunately, even when the early obvious fatigue effects are past the head-injured person will still need to manage his energy level carefully. He will need to plan to have extra rest periods if he has an unusual or demanding activity coming up. He will also need to be aware that it may take two or three days for him to recover from this activity.

Managing fatigue
Monitor activities
Ensure frequent rest periods, especially after tiring activities
Protect from well meaning friends
Communicate with rehabilitation staff

Poor concentration and attention

Problems with concentration are closely linked to tiredness, and probably have the same basic cause. When we talk about impaired concentration there are three different ways in which this will affect what the head-injured person can do.

Focused attention

The first is that he will find it hard to keep his attention focused on one thing. He will find it hard to concentrate on doing a rehabilitation exercise, for example, and ignore what is going on in the room around him. You will find that when you talk to him he is easily distracted and cannot ignore trivial movements or noises. Anything is likely to grab his attention, even things that you have not noticed. This is because while we focus our attention on what we are doing we are normally able to use part of our attention mechanism to keep track of what is going on around us. The head-injured person is unable to do this. For this reason the rehabilitation staff will usually try to treat him in a quiet room on his own, to reduce the number of things that might distract him. It is important that you also watch out for this. As an example, if he still needs to put all his attention into keeping his balance when he walks, talking to him at the same time is not the right thing to do!

Divided attention

The second, related, way in which the problem which the head-injured person has with concentrating will show is when he tries to divide his attention between two things at the same time. Normally we do this without thinking about it. For example, whenever we write down a telephone message, take notes during a lecture, or look after a child while listening to a friend talk, we are using this special skill. After a head injury the person does not have enough concentration to focus on one task, so it is not surprising that he cannot cope with two. The best way to help him through this stage is to arrange things so that he does not have to divide his attention between several sources. Try to restrict visitors to one at a time, for example.

Attention span

The third way in which poor attention is shown is in the length of time that the head-injured person is able to concentrate on a task —

the concentration span. In the early stages this can be as short as five minutes. The rehabilitation staff will take this into account, knowing that there is no point expecting him to stick at an exercise once he has exhausted his ability to concentrate. Family and friends need to understand too that he may be capable of doing something at one point in time, and then be unable to continue a short time later. The family should keep in mind how long the 'attention span' is, and not expect him to concentrate for longer than this. It is reassuring to know that the concentration span will get longer as the weeks go by. It is also important to remember that when a head-injured person is tired his concentration will be even worse. You can encourage him to plan his days so that the toughest jobs are tackled when he is fresh and alert. He also needs to be reassured that the right thing to do is to take rests, or have a sleep if he feels tired, rather than to try to finish what he is doing in one sitting and probably fail at it.

Problems of concentration
Difficulties with:
focused attention — ignoring distraction
divided attention — eg taking lecture notes
attention span — how long does concentration last?

Memory problems

It will be easier to understand how memory can go wrong after a head injury if you know the way that memory normally works. It is important to realize that it is not a simple one-stage system. There are several steps that have to be carried through. Before we can remember something we first have to notice it, or attend to it. Next we have to store it in the brain and it has to be stored in such a way that we can get it back later when we want to recall it. It then has to stay safe in storage, and lastly we have to be able to recall it when it is needed.

The next fact about 'normal' memory is that there are differences in the way memories are stored, depending on whether or not they contain information that we will try to get back to later. Not all of the things we have to remember every day have to be remembered for very long. A telephone number can be remembered for as long as it takes to make a call, but it may never be used again and so it can be forgotten safely. Other things we may never forget for as long as we live. This tells us that some memories are permanent and others only temporary. Things we have known for a long time, a childhood memory or words of our native language, are permanent memories which are unlikely to be lost, and which seem to be stored in the brain in a different way to new information. Things that we have known for a short time only, such as the name of a new acquaintance or a new address, are more easily forgotten. However, some temporary memories can later become permanent if conditions are right. This happens when we have a use for that memory and refer to it or recall it frequently. This regular use or exercise of a memory makes it more likely to endure and to eventually become a permanent memory. We all make use of this fact when we study. We know that if we rehearse something often enough we will be able to remember it when we need to. Of course the opposite is also true. If we make no use of newly learned information we will quickly forget it.

There is one other fact about how memory works which we need to understand in order to understand how a head injury can affect it. This is the concept of separate memory 'factories'. Memories of conversations, pictures, maps, or smells appear to be handled separately by the brain. For example, the parts of the brain that work together to remember faces are different from those that are used to remember the names that go with these faces. In the same way, different parts of the brain are used to remember maps or diagrams than are used to remember a poem.

Stages of memory
Attend
Store (different stores for different memories):
(a) for a short time (temporary memory)
(b) for later recall (long-term memory)
Remember:
(a) without any hints (recall)
(b) when a clue is given (recognition)

Memory is therefore a very complex system, and there are many different stages and parts of this system which can be affected by head injury. Often some parts are working well, while others are damaged. There is usually no problem recalling permanent memories which were laid down before the accident, but many head-injured people have difficulty laying down new memories in some or all of the memory 'factories'. Thus your relative or friend may be able to recall details of a family gathering that happened many years ago and that you had almost forgotten, but not be able to tell you what he had for lunch yesterday. It may be difficult for friends and relatives to understand this selective recall, and why the rehabilitation team is concerned about it. You will understand now, we hope, that recalling the family gathering does not mean that he has a good memory, but rather that his ability to lay down new memories is impaired but the ability to recall 'old' memories has not been affected.

We have not yet discussed the memory problem that head-injured persons are most likely to be concerned about. This is the memory gap around the accident. The head-injured person cannot remember what happened to him, or how it happened. Sometimes he will have no memory of things that happened for a while before the injury. He will also have another sort of memory loss for things that happened after the injury. Not only can he not remember the time that he was unconscious, but he cannot remember some of the time after he woke up, even though he may have spent this time apparently awake and talking with friends and family. These two sorts of memory loss are sometimes called retrograde amnesia and post-traumatic amnesia.

Retrograde amnesia

At the moment of injury the brain stops noticing and storing memories. This is why there is rarely any memory of the injury itself, although occasionally things happening up to the instant may be remembered. More usually the last clear memory of the head-injured person may be something that happened some minutes, hours, days, or occasionally months or even years before. Sometimes the person will remember a few things that fall within this time of otherwise total memory loss. Usually these memories are of special significance, such as a family wedding.

As he gets better he may remember a few more of the things that happened before the injury, but he is unlikely to remember everything. In particular he is unlikely to remember the instant of the injury itself. This is why it is pointless for him to waste energy trying to remember it, and why you do not need to worry about the emotional effect it might have on him if he does get this memory back. He can never remember the accident because he does not have that memory in his brain. The moment of impact interrupted the mechanism where the brain changes things that are experienced into a form which makes it possible for them to be remembered later. The things that happened immediately before and at the time of the impact did not have time to be changed into memories, so they can never be remembered.

Post-traumatic amnesia

Even after a fairly minor head injury there will be a time after the head-injured person has apparently 'woken up' which he will later be unable to remember. This time can range from a few seconds or minutes to days, weeks or months. During this period he may answer or ask questions, he may walk around, have a meal, or do other apparently 'awake' things, but because he is completely unable to remember them later we know that he was obviously not actually awake. It may help to understand this stage if you compare it to sleepwalking. We are not usually surprised that we do not remember things that happen while we are asleep. In the same way, do not expect your relative or friend to remember what happened during this stage. He has not woken up enough to have the ability to put things which happen into memory store.

Earlier we explained how it is unreasonable to expect a head-injured person to have a good memory if he is not able to attend to what goes on around him. Because problems with concentration and attention are so very common in the early days after the injury, memory problems are also very common at that time, and often improved concentration is accompanied by improved memory. When this does not happen it suggests that the breakdown is because he has problems storing memories in the brain, or maybe problems getting stored memories out again when he needs them.

Coping with a poor memory

The first step in dealing with a memory problem is to find out where the problem is. For this reason your relative or friend will have seen a neuro-psychologist, and you and the rehabilitation staff will know which parts of the system he can manage, and which parts have been affected by the injury. Memory retraining will make use of this information. If the problem is in putting things into memory store, for example, a head-injured person will be taught ways of doing this more effectively. The same applies to problems with retrieval, that is, of getting something out of memory when you want to. Or it may be that the 'memory factory' that handles words is still able to work, but the one that deals with pictures is rather useless. In these cases, exercises will concentrate on teaching him how to use the good 'word factory' to remember pictures, by translating the important parts of these pictures into words.

However, any kind of memory retraining is very labour intensive, and for many people it is not effective. In contrast, the technique of making memory 'external' gives immediate success. Making memory external simply means that pressure is taken off the brain by writing down things that have to be remembered. By using notepads, by making lists, by using calendars and diaries, a head-injured person can greatly increase the capacity of his memory. The rehabilitation team can give advice on ways that will work best for individual cases. In situations where it is very important that nothing is forgotten, for example, a pocket tape recorder may be more useful than trying to take notes. It may never be possible to make faulty memory into fault-free memory, but by limiting the number of things that the head-injured person forgets he can regain a degree of control over his life. He is now in charge of the memory problem rather than the other way round.

Writing things down is an excellent way of coping with a poor memory. It does not hinder recovery.

You as the care-giver can help him to establish a routine to make sure that looking in the diary, or checking the calendar, become part of daily life. You can also help by reassuring him that managing the memory problem in this way, by taking much of the load off internal memory, is the most effective way of helping that memory to work.

Lack of insight

Insight is being realistic about how well you are able to do things. When your head-injured friend or family member lacks insight he cannot appreciate the way in which other people react to what he does, and because of this he does not see any need to alter how he acts. This ability to judge the effect of what we do and say on other people, and to use this knowledge to modify our behaviour, is controlled by the front parts of the brain behind the forehead. When this part of the brain is not working efficiently the person may genuinely believe that there is nothing wrong with him, or he may focus on a minor consequence of the accident, such as a stiff knee, and deny that he has any other problems. Of course, as long as he does not see that there is any need for it he will be unlikely to make much progress in rehabilitation. It will be hard to convince him that he should work at overcoming a concentration problem, for example, if he is sure that his concentration is as good as it ever was.

Not only does lack of insight make it hard for the rehabilitation staff, but it is also hard for families and care-givers. Because he is unable to appreciate the consequences of what he does, his behaviour may be impulsive and often potentially dangerous. For instance, he may insist on driving a car or riding a motor cycle, even though the rehabilitation team have forbidden this because his reaction times are too slow for him to be safe, and because his ability to judge the distance and speed of oncoming traffic is poor. Try to avoid this kind of situation from developing by removing the motor cycle, for example, or by anticipating when he might want to go out, and offering to drive him yourself. Lack of insight is most common in the early days after a severe head injury, and in most cases the person will also find it hard to concentrate and will have a poor memory. Because of this, it is usually possible to distract him if he attempts to do something where he or others may be harmed. However, you need to be quite vigilant, and you should also make sure that you have reliable helpers to take your place so that your relative or friend is not left alone if you need to go out.

If the head-injured person's insight is poor
He might deny that there are problems
He may not see the need for rehabilitation
He may endanger others by his actions

The carer must be very vigilant
The carer must enlist 'minders' when they go out

Insight will improve as the head-injured person gets better, but this is unlikely to happen overnight. One day he might be quite realistic, and the next deny that he has any problems. You can help by making him aware of what he can and cannot do. Discuss the problems with the rehabilitation team, and support them in their efforts to promote realism.

Slowed reactions

Because the brain does not have the normal amount of energy, the head-injured person will be unable to do things as quickly or as efficiently as he could before the accident. This happens with mental as well as physical activities. You will also find that he can take much longer to do even fairly simple automatic activities, such as eating or cleaning his teeth. He will usually be unaware that he has been so slow, because he is doing these tasks as quickly as his slowed-down brain will allow. Do not fall into the trap of thinking that he is being deliberately obstructive, or trying to get you upset because you will be late for whatever appointment you have arranged for him. Make sure that you plan ahead, and arrange to start getting him ready several hours before the deadline.

When he has to carry out some complex activity such as making a decision he may work so slowly that he does not finish the task at all, because by the time he gets to considering the alternatives he has usually forgotten what they all are. You must make allowances for this. In the early stages after the head injury he needs to be protected from the physical danger which can result from coping with dangerous machinery, or from driving a motor vehicle while he still has slowed reactions. The second way you can help your head-injured relative or friend is to protect him from the need to cope with complex problems. The rehabilitation team will help you work out how you can break up these problems into smaller parts that are easier for the head-injured person to cope with.

Headache

Headaches occur frequently after even quite mild head injury. This book cannot replace the medical advice that you will seek if your friend or family member is bothered by headaches. They can have many causes, and your doctor will need to investigate these. However, one of the most common causes, particularly when headaches occur for the first time some months after injury, is stress or tension. Often the headaches show that the person is trying to do too much, and disappear when the activity that has brought on the headache is stopped. In other cases they can be a sign that he is becoming anxious and concerned about himself, his job, or his family life. A stress management programme is often useful, and he will usually find that when he has mastered some relaxation techniques he will be able to reduce the intensity of the headache, if not eliminate it completely.

Emotional ups and downs

In the early stages after injury there can be one of two emotional 'reactions' which are seen regardless of what happens round the head-injured person. At one extreme he may appear to be very happy, unconcerned by his plight, and never troubled by sadness even when told news which would normally distress him. At the other extreme he may show no emotion at all. He may appear uncaring, unmoved, unloving, and untouchable, almost as though his feelings have been lost. This is because one of the consequences of head injury can be that the person expresses emotion differently, or reacts differently in emotional situations. The early stage, whether of extreme elation or complete loss of feeling, is usually replaced by a stage where emotions appear to be running wild. There may be swings of mood, perhaps from a real 'high' to a desperate 'low'. Emotions not normally part of the personality may make themselves more obvious.

Our familiar emotional reactions are built up through long experience. The brain makes sense of our emotional experience so that we react in the appropriate way. While growing up we learn to recognize signs of fear, anger, and other emotions in our own body. These are things that we do not think about doing, they just happen automatically. We know for certain, without any hesitation, that we are angry, happy, sad or elated. A head injury can alter this way of experiencing the world. Ordinary everyday experiences may suddenly have the potential to unsettle him or to make him feel uncomfortable. Crowds of people, the noise and bustle of the street, and the babble of noisy places may all be experienced as unpleasant or even frightening. Emotions may be experienced in a confusing way, so that he is unsure just what he is feeling. The ability to gauge the emotional reactions of others, to tell by their faces if they are happy or sad, can be impaired by the injury.

Very often the person loses the ability to control emotional reactions such as tears or laughter. Sometimes this shows itself in not being able to stop one of these reactions once it has started, long after the emotion associated with it has been spent. Sometimes the tears or laughter are triggered by an inappropriate (or even no) emotion. He may be unable to control tears whenever he feels excited, even if this excitement is brought on by a favourite sports team scoring a goal. Sometimes any attempt to concentrate may bring on uncontrollable laughter, no matter how serious he feels at the time. For some head-injured people tears and laughter seem to be severed from feelings, and occur for no apparent reason. These reactions can be embarrassing for family and friends as well as for the head-injured person. He will need reassurance from you that you understand his behaviour, and that you will explain to those around if he is unable to do this himself. It is also important to remember that, as with all the other effects of the accident, ability to control emotion will fluctuate with fatigue. Make sure that he is rested if he has to cope with situations which could trigger tears or laughter.

Other emotional responses which can be affected by head injury are irritability and aggression. This behaviour is very common when the person is first waking up, and the response may be to lash out with a fist at anyone within range. He may be unable to express feelings in any way other than aggression. As an example, he may grasp your hand, which you know is because he wants you to stay with him, but then he either squeezes your hand so hard that it hurts, or else pinches your flesh or attempts to twist your finger. This is as much out of conscious control as the vocabulary that he may use at this time, which is often full of swear words. You need to realize that the aggression and bad language are not directed specifically at you. You need also to realize that this is not something that you can 'talk over' and settle when he is better, because this period is one which he will not be able to remember later on.

Even after he has recovered enough to remember things that happen to him from day to day, he may be easily irritated by rather trivial things, and aggression can still be a problem. If he is difficult at home you may be hurt to learn from the rehabilitation team that his behaviour when he is with them is very good. He does not lose his temper, he does not shout and swear, and he does not throw things. There is a very simple explanation for this. Paradoxical as it may seem, he behaves badly in your company because he feels safe with you and he knows that you love him too. He does not feel this way with any of the people at the rehabilitation centre and he expends considerable energy controlling the aggression, because he knows that if he 'blows up' there he is likely to be asked to leave. He can relax once he gets home, and in a very real sense you are the safety valve. You need to talk about this problem with the team. Although the head-injured person will not be able to cope with a standard anger management course at this stage, the team may be able to help him, and they certainly will be able to teach you how to manage these moods. Obviously if you do not discuss this with the team they can have no idea that anger is a problem. It may also help you to ride out this stage if you can accept that the behaviour of the head-injured person is not a personal attack on you, and that things really will get better as time goes on.

We need to describe one more emotional response which typically occurs rather late in the recovery cycle. It is quite natural for a head-injured person to become depressed as he gets better and gains more insight. With insight comes the realization of how many losses there have been, loss of individual freedom, loss of mobility, loss of skills, and perhaps mental, physical, and emotional losses. The depressed mood is therefore a realistic reaction to the many losses that he has experienced.

This mood of despondency may come and go over days, weeks, or months. The person may express feelings of frustration, anger, or despair, and may talk of ending it all. If you are worried that he might do himself an injury or worse, then talk to your own doctor or to someone from the rehabilitation team, and make sure that it is checked out to your satisfaction. Note, however, that an emotional reaction of this sort, which can be alarming to family and friends, is a positive sign of recovery. You cannot feel blue about your problems without first knowing what they are. This recognition is vital to the success of continuing rehabilitation. You can help the head-injured person to understand that his depression is a positive sign that he is getting better; if left to himself he may decide that he is getting worse as he feels so much worse. This would only exacerbate his already anxious and confused state, and he may worry about all the awful things that must be happening inside his head.

Understanding and accepting depression or anxiety as a natural and healthy reaction allows the rehabilitation to proceed in a positive way. Depression viewed this way is a step on the path to recovery.

Stages in emotional control

Early stage:
either over-happy or no emotions

Middle stage:
over-reaction
irritability
aggression
inappropriate tears/laughter

Later stage:
ability to control moods with strangers
depressed
may still over-react

Changes in sexuality

The sexuality of the head-injured person can be disturbed because of physical, psychological, or social changes. Importence is a common problem, but one which they may feel unwilling or unable to talk about with the rehabilitation staff, or with relatives or friends. In the early stages fatigue will be a contributing factor, and so time may bring a solution. However, even in these early stages he should talk over the problem with a doctor, if you can persuade him to do this.

Psychological changes can arise because of the way head-injured people can see themselves following the accident. Loss, scarring, or paralysis of limbs can seriously affect the self-image, leading to problems in dealing with social or sexual partners. Less obvious losses such as a change in job status can also lead to a loss of confidence in social situations, or a loss of self-esteem.

In social situations he may unwittingly break unwritten rules. For example he may infringe on 'personal space' by moving too close when he is talking to someone, and nobody likes to feel pressured in this way. Neither are people likely to be impressed if the head-injured person forgot to clean his teeth or take a shower. He may appear forward, touch people when he ought not to, or make jokes which are in bad taste. This type of behaviour can be seen as sexually provocative or out of place. Social rule-breaking is common after a head injury, and it comes about because the person no longer has the ability to judge how the things he does are affecting other people.

If your friend or relative behaves in a sexually inappropriate way you can help him to change by pointing out why the things that he does are unacceptable. If possible, show him a way of doing things or a way of expressing his feelings which is more acceptable. Do not expect quick results because the problem has its basis in impaired brain function. You may feel embarrassed and unable to talk about his behaviour with the head-injured person. In this case discuss the problem with whichever member of the rehabilitation team you feel most comfortable with. He or she will understand, and will also be able to talk with the head-injured person about your worries.

If you are caring for a head-injured person who lived independently before the accident it is important that you allow him some independence in your new living arrangements. Too often parents fall into the trap of treating their adult children as having no sexual feelings, or having no need of privacy. As he gets better he will want to spend some of his time alone with friends, and this should be respected. Unfortunately the old friends may not continue to visit, and he will find it hard to meet new friends. Throughout this book we have stressed the importance of professional counselling. This is a time when he needs help. But it is also a time when you as the care-giver could benefit from a sympathetic ear, and benefit from advice about coping with an adult child or friend who is no longer able to manage his own sexual life.

Case histories

Samuel

The Friday before Samuel was due to go back to school Mr Smith called to see him. Samuel's parents had both thanked him already for his neighbourly action in looking after the lad, and he had heard the good news that the leg was stable enough for him to get up and about again. Mr Smith was puffing a bit by the time he got to the drive, carrying a large packet of barley sugar as a back-to-school present. It was then that, for the first time, Samuel's parents heard that he had been knocked out in the crash, and that it had been 'some time' before he woke up and started crying. They wondered if this would make a difference to his fitness to return to school, and decided to make a visit to the family doctor to talk about it.

The doctor asked about Samuel's behaviour, and his moods, and asked Samuel how much he remembered of the accident. The parents learned that rather than a subconscious 'repression' of events, the boy's memory gaps for things that happened before and after his fall were because he had been knocked out. When he heard that Samuel was still sleeping a lot, and still complained of headaches and sore eyes, the doctor advised his parents to keep him home from school for another three weeks, or until he was able to stay awake all day.

Samuel's mother was worried about asking her employer for more time off work to look after him, and eventually it was decided to send him to stay with his grandparents at their home on the coast. This proved to be an excellent decision. There was no stereo, no hustle and no bustle, and the loudest noise in the house was the ticking of the clock on the mantelpiece. Grandpa played board games with him at the drop of a hat, grandma made sure he had a regular sleep period during the afternoon, and the three of them strolled along the waterfront every evening so Samuel had the exercise he needed. By the end of the first week he did not have one headache all day, and there were no tears or tantrums.

Jonas

Although Jonas would not admit it to his parents, he revelled in being with them at first. He had gone home on a Friday evening, and it was luxury to sleep in his own bed, and to sleep in till he awoke in the morning, and not when the rehabilitation staff needed him to have his shower. He also realized that he had forgotten what a good cook his mother was. She in turn was surprised that he ate everything she put in front of him, even broccoli! Before his accident he would never have allowed broccoli on his plate and she had not intended to serve him any, but he insisted that he wanted some, and appeared to eat it with relish. The first weekend was pleasant. Jonas had a drive to the beach with his friends, and spent most of the next day dozing on a hammock in the garden.

Stephen, who was to provide his attendant care, arrived promptly at nine o'clock on Monday morning to drive Jonas to his out-patient appointment. Jonas was not as prompt. He had refused to get out of bed when his mother had roused him, and was still abusing her roundly for disturbing him when Stephen came in. After that, and after talking it over with Suzy, the accident insurers agreed that Stephen should come an hour earlier to get Jonas up, and to oversee his shower and breakfast.

By the end of the first month Jonas had learned to dress himself in track-suits without help, and to put on shoes with velcro fastenings. However, he could not yet manage buttons or shoelaces, and still had to be really careful to work out which was the front and which the back of his clothes before he put them on. Cooking lessons had progressed faster, but he still needed to be reminded to put on the timer when he put things under the grill, and if the occupational therapy department had not had a kettle which switched off automatically he would have burnt out an element every time he tried to make himself a cup of coffee.

He was amazed to find how tiring he found it to concentrate during this rehabilitation, and would not admit even to Stephen that he often got to the end of the session and could not remember what he had been doing. He was so tired by the time that he got home that he often fell asleep at the dining table, and his father had to help him off to bed.

There was a crisis some weeks later. Stephen had been delayed and did not collect him on time from the rehabilitation centre. This took them into rush-hour traffic, and Jonas became more and more agitated. Eventually he jumped from the car, yelling that it would be quicker to walk! By the time Stephen had managed to find somewhere to leave the car safely, Jonas was out of sight. Stephen ran along the footpath and when he rounded a corner saw a small crowd gathered round his charge, who was in the firm grip of a rather large policeman. By this time Jonas was incoherent and crying, and it took a visit to the police station, a lengthy interview, and the arrival of the doctor from the rehabilitation unit, before the police were convinced that Jonas was not under the influence of alcohol or drugs, and did not need to be charged with disorderly behaviour!

Pauline

It was half-way through the next afternoon when Pauline woke up. Her husband had taken the day off school to be with her, and he had begun to be concerned that maybe he should not let her sleep so long, so he was relieved to see her stir and open her eyes. She had to sit on the edge of the bed for some minutes when she tried to get up, as the room was spinning round her. It was not until this dizzy spell had passed that she realized it was odd that John was not at school. She could not believe it was the weekend already, and was relieved to hear that it was only one day after she had gone to sleep. She was not quite so relieved to hear how late it was, or to be reminded of her sojourn at the emergency department. It was then that she remembered the court case, and tried to insist that she had to get to work to sort it out. John was astonished that she appeared to have totally forgotten her colleague's visit to the hospital, and his assurance that he would deal with the case. Pauline was shattered, as she did not remember this visit at all, let alone the conversation. Her first reaction was that for some reason John was attempting to trick her so that she would stay home, and it was only after she had phoned her law firm that she realized that it was *her* memory that was at fault. She put down the telephone and burst into tears.

6
Some specific consequences

Some or all of the after-effects which we talked about in the last chapter can be seen in anyone who has had a closed head injury, whether it was mild or severe. You will remember that in Chapter 2 we described how in this sort of injury damage occurs to widespread areas of the brain because of the distortion and twisting which occurs. Penetrating injuries or blood clots on the other hand cause more localized damage, with different effects. These often look like the results of a stroke, perhaps with paralysis of one side of the body or loss of speech. Often both sorts of damage are present at the same time, which makes them more difficult to deal with.

Arms, legs, walking, and balance

All animals, ourselves included, depend on strong, well-coordinated arms and legs and a good sense of balance when we are walking or climbing. Humans have the extra burden of balancing upright and controlling skilled movements of the hands and arms. This is mostly achieved automatically, without giving it a thought. It is no wonder that injury, by accident or disease, can have so profound an effect on this complex function.

Weakness

As we mentioned in Chapter 2, damage to one side of the brain commonly results in weakness of the other side of the body, a 'hemiplegia' or 'half-paralysis'. Many people will be aware of this from seeing what happens after a stroke. The hand is usually more affected than the elbow and shoulder and will often remain weak and clumsy when there has been good recovery elsewhere. Although it may be difficult to put much power into a movement, the muscles themselves are strong, and in many cases stiff or 'spastic', so that they resist any attempt to move the joints they work on. Reflexes may be very active, so that if a muscle is stretched quickly, for example by putting the foot down on the floor and bending the ankle up, it may contract repeatedly and set up a juddering movement, called 'clonus'. Over-action of spastic muscles may pull a joint into an abnormal position. If it is allowed to stay in this position the joint may stiffen (a 'contracture' of the joint) and be a serious handicap to getting function back.

The head injuries which result in paralysis of this sort are often those where there has been a bruise or blood clot pressing on one side of the brain. In many cases of severe head injury the damage is more widespread and affects the deeper parts of the brain, producing a different picture. Early after the injury the legs are stiff and straight, with the toes pointed; the arms are stiff as well, and either straight or sharply bent at the elbow. In this position the joints may become contracted and stiff and great care is needed to prevent this. Later, when some recovery has taken place, one arm and both legs usually remain weak and spastic, the other arm often being nearly normal. There are, however, many variations in this pattern.

Loss of power in arms and legs
Hemiplegia:
localized damage to one side of the brain
one side of the body affected

Three limbs affected — *'triplegia'*
widespread damage, including deeper parts of the brain
one arm and both legs affected

Coordination and balance

The ability to coordinate movements of the arms and legs comes from another system in the brain. In a stroke, when the damage to the brain is localized, little clumsiness may accompany the weakness. Trauma usually produces more widespread damage and coordination is likely to be affected as well as strength, so that there is both weakness and clumsiness. Occasionally the coordination system only is affected, and then there is clumsiness with nearly normal strength.

Balance and control of body posture are other aspects of coordination and are needed as soon as we get up from a lying position. In the early stages of recovery after a severe injury, problems will therefore begin as soon as the patient tries to sit up. Usually their head will fall forward or to one side and without support their body will slump down. In time muscle tone will improve, they will be able to hold their head up and then sit on their own. As the proper tone in the trunk and leg muscles is re-learned, they will be ready to stand and later walk.

At an early stage two other systems need to come into action. The first system makes it possible to recognize what position your body is in and how it relates to the world around you. Fit people take this for granted; they know instantly which way is up and with a glance they can tell what is around them and what they could reach out for and lean on for support. After a severe brain injury this ability is often lost. Fit people find it difficult to appreciate how frightening this can be; it is said that it is like living one's life on a roller-coaster. Therefore the head-injury patient needs to relearn these necessary skills, so that each day he can become more aware of where his body and limbs are in space and he can learn to estimate what is around him.

The other vital system is inner ear balance, the 'vestibular' system. The balance organs are enclosed in dense bone at the base of the skull, alongside the organs of hearing. They are very small and delicate and easily upset. Even after mild head injuries there are often balance problems, which show up as a feeling of dizziness and spinning, usually when the head is moved suddenly. Severe injuries may put them out of action altogether, and the lack of information about balance may make it very difficult to sit securely and to make the first moves towards walking.

Co-ordination
Needs strength, recognition of posture and control

Balance
Needs coordination

Needs information from: balance organ in ears
                                    vision
                                    experience and thought

Posture
Needs balance, and ability to sustain effort
Necessary before beginning to walk

Much of early rehabilitation will be taken up with these problems. In the stage of coma the physiotherapists will make sure that joints are kept moving and at the same time protected from the strain that abnormal muscle pull can cause in an unconscious patient. As consciousness returns, they will start to get the patient sitting up in a chair, at first needing help to hold their head up, then onto a tilting bed to accustom them slowly to being upright, and at length standing. In this way they will redevelop their skills of knowing where they are in space and controlling posture.

Walking

In getting as far as this, they will have taken a few uncertain steps from bed to chair; now they can start in earnest to re-learn to walk. This is one of the major goals of recovery, a sign of achievement and independence. To begin with, support will be needed, first from the therapists and then from wheeled frames that steady the balance and take some of the weight on the arms, and then from sticks. Splints may be needed to support the knee joint or to hold the foot in a good position.

How far the recovery of walking goes will depend mostly on the initial severity of the injury. Some will walk much as they did before. At the other extreme, they may only be able to take a few steps and prefer to use a wheelchair to get around outside their home. The best measure of success is how good their function is, rather than how close to normal they look. This is an important point because some people become obsessed by their desire to walk and reject practical aids to function such as sticks and wheelchairs.

Everyday living skills

At the same time as posture, balance and mobility are being regained, the occupational therapists will be using the re-learned skills to get the patient back to the business of everyday living. Practice eating, washing and all the other simple activities of everyday life will teach him to recognize where he is, what is going on around him and how he relates to the world. Later their teaching will extend to improving coordination and manual skills, to writing and using a typewriter or computer.

Regaining the skills of everyday life
Using re-learned coordination and balance to cope with
  activities of daily life
Improving coordination by using manual skills

Spontaneous movements

Some people develop troublesome spontaneous movements after a head injury, which you may hear called 'chorea' or 'ballismus'. Usually just one arm is affected and either at rest or in the middle of a movement it will suddenly make a quite inappropriate movement, sometimes quite violently. The arm may move as whole or just the hand or fingers may be affected. The cause is damage to the deep central parts of the brain. Medication may help to control the movements, or occasionally an operation on the brain, similar to the operation done for Parkinson's disease, may be advised.

Post-traumatic epilepsy

Diagnosing post-traumatic epilepsy

In Chapter 2 we saw that damage to some parts of the brain can result in scarring which makes the electrical activity of the brain unstable and leads to epilepsy. This shows itself by 'fits', or to use a less unpleasant term, 'seizures'. There are several sorts of seizure. Most easily recognized are the major seizures, in which consciousness is lost and there is to-and-fro shaking of the arms and legs. In other sorts of seizure consciousness may be lost without much else to see, sometimes for quite a short time, perhaps for less than a minute. They may remain standing or their legs may collapse under them. During the seizure or when it has just finished they may do things which are quite well organized but inappropriate, like walking round in a circle or repeating meaningless words. After this they may be confused for a while. Sometimes the seizures may be even less noticeable, described as just 'shutting off' for a few moments.

Usually the family will have little doubt that something abnormal is happening, though it may be difficult to be sure when there have been episodes when they just 'shut off'. When they tell the doctor about it, making a diagnosis of the nature and the cause of the seizure will depend very much on a clear description of what happened, and it will be very helpful if the family carefully observe the details, and preferably write them down.

Usually an electroencephalogram (EEG) is done to help to diagnose the cause of the seizures. We mentioned the EEG in Chapter 2; it is a recording of the minute electric currents that the brain produces, picked up by wires resting on the scalp. In many cases there are well marked irregularities which make the diagnosis definite and give some idea of where in the brain the trouble is coming from. Note, however, that the EEG is not the last word, and in some cases where there are definite seizures it is not abnormal. It may be possible to locate an abnormal area in the brain which is causing the seizures in an MR scan. Again, we talked about MR scans in Chapter 2. They are a very powerful tool in locating damaged areas of the brain.

Post-traumatic epilepsy
'Major' seizures with convulsions
'Minor' seizures, 'shutting off'

Diagnosis of seizure
Requires a good description of what happens
EEG recordings, which may not be abnormal
MR scans, sometimes valuable

Treatment

When a definite diagnosis of post-traumatic epilepsy has been made, 'anti-convulsant' medication will usually be prescribed. This works by reducing the tendency of the brain to respond to the irritation of the brain from the scarring. If it is to be useful at all it must be taken regularly all the time, as a protection, a sort of insurance policy. There is no point in taking it irregularly, and in fact this may do harm. If for any reason it has to be stopped, it must be tailed off gradually over two or three weeks — stopping it abruptly may set off a seizure.

When the medication is started it will be necessary to check that the dose is correct — different people need different amounts. This will be judged by whether it is effective in stopping the seizures and whether there are any unpleasant side effects. Usually the amount of anticonvulsant in the blood will be measured, every week or two to begin with and then, when the dose is stabilized, every few months.

What is the chance of post-traumatic epilepsy occurring?

The most important factor in determining the chance of post-traumatic epilepsy is the sort of injury that there was. In general, injury to the surface of the brain is important, and with open wounds of the brain the risk is high. In closed injuries bruising of the brain and blood clots are also potent causes. As a very rough guide, an open wound damaging five or so square centimetres of the surface of the brain, and a bruise of roughly the same size in a closed injury, will result in a one in five chance of epilepsy. With more details, the doctor may be able to give a more reliable estimate of the risk.

The seizures can start in the first days or weeks after the accident, or can first appear five years or more later. Often the first one is pre-cipitated by alcohol, loss of sleep or excessive fatigue. The risk lessens as time passes. If there has been no seizure after three years, the risk is less than a quarter of the original risk, and at ten years it is probably no greater than the risk in the population as a whole.

Can post-traumatic epilepsy be prevented?

The first measure to prevent epilepsy is to make sure that wounds are treated properly. If the wound is cleaned thoroughly and all damaged tissue removed it will heal smoothly and the risk will be reduced.

The second measure which is sometimes advised is to give anti-convulsant medication even though there has been no sign of a seizure. It is possible that if the medication is given immediately after the injury the damaged area never gets a chance to destabilize the brain around it, and that if the drugs are discontinued after a year or so the risk is over. It is fair to say that it has not yet been shown that this is the case. However, many doctors feel that epilepsy is so disabling that if there is a reasonable chance of reducing the risk it is worth the inconvenience of taking medication for a year. This is a choice which needs to be dis-cussed with the patient and family to decide on the merits of each case — how big the risk is and how they feel about taking the precaution.

Treating post-traumatic epilepsy
Medication should be started:
when it is certain that seizures are occurring

Medication may be chosen:
if the risk of epilepsy is high

If medication is being taken:
it must be taken regularly
dosage and blood levels must be checked regularly

If medication is stopped for any reason:
it must be tailed off gradually

Stopping anti-convulsant medication

When there is a question of post-traumatic epilepsy, there will probably need to be a review of the situation a year after the injury. If seizures have occurred, either before or after starting medication, anti-convulsants will need to be continued, with a review of the dosage.

If there have been no seizures but medication has been given with the aim of preventing them the decision may be more difficult. If we discontinue medication we will be waiting to see if a seizure occurs and whether the policy has been successful. For someone who is still in hospital or in rehabilitation this does not pose a great risk. For someone who is back to near normal activity, perhaps driving a car, the decision poses difficult problems. Should they continue to drive, or go swimming or sailing, accepting that they may have a seizure in a place of danger? Should they avoid some activities until they know whether they are at serious risk of epilepsy? If so, how long do they have to wait?

There are no easy answers to these questions. The patient's lifestyle is one major factor. What is their work, how much do they depend on using their car? Are they able to come to a reasonable decision about the problem or has their judgment been affected by the accident? Another major factor is the actual risk of having a seizure. As we mentioned before, we can get an estimate of this from the nature of the injury. This can be strengthened by information from an EEG. If this is definitely abnormal it can be a good reason to continue with medication. Unfortunately if it is normal it cannot be taken as ruling out the risk of epilepsy.

When as much of the information as possible has been assembled a final decision must be made by patient and doctor, with the help of the partner or a close relative. If it is decided to discontinue, the dosage must be reduced slowly over two or three weeks, and definite safety rules agreed on for the next six months or so, depending on the estimate of risk. If medication is to be continued, another date for review may be set in perhaps a year.

Discontinuing anti-convulsant drugs also becomes an issue when they have been started or continued because of seizures and a number of years have passed without any further evidence of epilepsy. There is no doubt that in some people the tendency to have seizures does diminish with the years. All the evidence possible of the activity of the epilepsy should be gathered and a decision taken, as before, in the light of this and the patient's lifestyle. Again, there are no easy answers.

> **Stopping medication**
> *Making the decision:*
> if they have never had seizures but have taken medication
>   to prevent them
> if they have had seizures but with medication none for
>   several years
>
> *The decision will depend on:*
> the risk of having more fits: your doctor can give you
>   advice about this on the basis of the facts of the injury
>   and on tests such as EEG
> what effect another fit would have: danger at work,
>   driving, social effects

Language and communication

When we use language, either to take in information or to express ourselves, we depend on a group of several separate but closely linked
centres in the brain, in most people in its left half. Depending on
where the damage is, each of the skills of listening and understanding,
talking, reading or writing can be separately affected by injury to the
brain, though usually there is a mixture of more than one defect. The
result is called 'dysphasia' if speech is still present to some degree,
'aphasia' if there is no speech at all. If the problem is with understanding speech, it is a 'receptive dysphasia'; if with producing speech, an
'expressive dysphasia'. There are other less important terms, such as
'nominal dysphasia' where the problem is in remembering names.

When we have something to communicate, we need to speak or
write. Making the sounds which consist of speech involves the control
of breathing and of the muscles of the voice box (the 'larynx') and the
throat. The parts of the brain responsible for this (centres in the
'medulla' and 'brain stem') are linked to the language centres but quite
separate from them. These centres are commonly damaged in more
severe injuries, with 'dysarthria' when there is still some speech possible and 'anarthria' when there is none. Again, writing may not be
possible if there is paralysis of the arm.

Understanding speech after a head injury

When your family member or friend begins to wake up after a head
injury you would expect them to be confused and muddled, with none

of the language centres working properly. As they become more alert it may become plain that part of the communication process is lagging behind in the recovery. Though they appear wide awake there might be no response at all even to simple commands such as 'put out your hand'. More often they would respond to simpler requests but not complicated ones — there would be a 'receptive dysphasia'. As recovery occurs it may become plain that they are having most problems with particular parts of speech, such as recognizing proper names.

You will appreciate that if they are to benefit from rehabilitation they need to regain the ability to take in the messages and instructions that they are given. Intensive work with the speech and language therapist is essential and other members of the rehabilitation team will not be able to get far with their work until the patient has regained some basic communication skills.

Speaking and communicating after a head injury

When damage has occurred to the areas of the brain responsible for producing speech, resulting in an 'expressive dysphasia', the effect is usually obvious. They may not produce any words at all, there may be nonsense words or proper words right out of context. There may be fluent sentences which have no meaning. Most often to begin with there may be a 'yes' or a 'no' which is reasonably appropriate. As recovery occurs the structure of sentences improves and words are used more correctly. In some cases where the damage has been more severe particular problems with naming, grammar, and sentence structure may persist and need long-term speech therapy. These problems are often accompanied by corresponding difficulties with written communication.

In some cases it is the actual production of the sounds of speech that prevents communication — the 'dysarthria' that is often seen after severe injuries. The choice of words and the sentence structure may be satisfactory, but the right sounds cannot be produced. There may be reduced force and energy, so that only a whisper can be produced, or reduced modulation so that the cadences of speech are lost and words are produced in a rhythmless monotone. Some elements of speech may not be pronounced properly and particular vowels or consonants may be distorted. In the worst cases no speech at all may be possible.

The techniques of speech therapy will be able to improve the speech of most people with dysarthria of this sort. In a few in which the condition is severe or when there is no speech at all aids such as electronic communicators and hand held word processors will make a tremendous difference and give the patient back the ability to communicate with the people around them.

When your friend or relative has problems of this sort you will need to keep in close touch with the speech and language therapist who is working with them. The therapist will tell you how to help him to make himself understood, and how to make it easier for him to understand what you are saying to him.

There are two important points to remember if people do have language problems after a head injury. The first is that though they can't express themselves, perhaps not even say any words, they may well be able to understand most of what is said to them. Because of this, you should always act as if they do understand. This will prevent situations arising where thoughtless visitors make hurtful comments to which they can't respond.

The second point to remember is that language used to express emotion seems to be handled by special parts of the brain, different from those ordinarily used for speech. This may have been less affected by the injury, so that if the head-injured person becomes upset and emotional words may break out. Unfortunately they are often aggressive or swear words, and this may distress people around him who don't understand what is happening. Remember that not being able to express themselves is even more disturbing to them than it is to you, and that it is their high level of frustration which is evoking the words.

If communication is a problem
Speak slowly and clearly
Use questions that only need 'yes' or 'no' to answer
Keep sentences simple
Always act as if they understand what you say
Remember that they may understand more than you think

Coping with the world around us

Just as damage to some parts of the brain can affect our understanding of what we hear and our ability to express ourselves by talking, in a similar way damage to other parts affects the way we see the world around us and how we find our way about it. Again, just as in most people the left side of the brain is concerned with language, the right side is more concerned with this ability.

Understanding what we see and reacting to the world around us

By the time we have passed childhood we have established many 'seeing' skills which we no longer have to think about. We are able to tell, for example, that a table is square, though when we see it at an angle it looks like a squashed rectangle. We can tell where it is and can reach out and touch it, or walk round it without bumping into it. Without being aware that we are working out a problem we can tell how far away a car is, what speed it is travelling at, and where to move to get out of its way.

These skills are linked to the ability to know where our body and arms and legs are in space and what position they are in. When we reach out to touch the table, we know where our hand is and how it is moving towards its target. We find this out not by sight only — we could find it in the dark — but by fitting together information from our joints and muscles and comparing it with the plan we made in our mind when we first saw and located the table.

In some people who have had a head injury, it may be difficult to use these automatic skills. In the most severe instances they may completely ignore one side of their body. They see nothing to that side. They may have no idea of what their position is, whether they are sitting safely or about to fall off that edge of their chair, or whether on that side there is their bed, the wall or empty space.

As recovery occurs the complete failure to recognize one side of the body changes to 'neglect' or 'inattention' — they may not notice something on that side, but will see it if it is pointed out to them. Later still, they will notice things automatically but be slow to respond. The same improvement will occur with coordination of the affected side of the body. To begin with they may not use the arm and leg on that side at all. It may distress their family to see them dressed with only the good arm properly in their pyjama jacket, and the other arm and leg bare. As they improve, they will probably remain clumsy on one side and liable to walk into the side of doorways and bump into people in the street.

It is often difficult for family and friends to understand this neglect and failure to respond on one side. In the early stages they should be careful to be on the 'good' side, where the patient can see and react to them, and concentrate on what they are saying. Anything that they need to use should be put there. Later it may be useful to approach from the 'bad' side to encourage a response.

As they improve, their family should be prepared for them to be clumsy, drop cups and to bump into doorways. They may find difficulty in using scissors, which need coordinated movements, or eating with a knife and fork, which depend on both hands working together. If these things are difficult, be patient and allow them extra time to do them. Try not to draw attention to the mess they are making, and never take over and do it yourself. They will feel bad enough about not being able to use their arm very well, without this extra blow to their self respect. You will feel better about sitting back and letting them make a hash of things if you remember that the only way they are going to improve is to be allowed to keep trying to do things for themselves.

The world around us when half of it is missing:
stand and speak on the good side
later, encourage the bad side
be patient when they are clumsy
think of their self-respect

Other senses: taste and smell, sight, body temperature

Taste and smell

Most of the enjoyment we get from food is in its aroma, coming from the kitchen while it is being prepared and then on our plate. We perceive this almost entirely with our sense of smell, because our tongue and palate taste only sweet, sour, and salt. Smells are recognized by an area of special nerve cells in the roof of the nose, connected through a thin plate of bone to the brain immediately above. These nerves are easily torn, partly or completely, and the sense of smell will then be impaired or lost. The only taste detected then will be from the tongue and plate, the tastes of sweet, sour, and salt. Rarely these tastes too can be lost, either from damage to the nerves to the tongue or to the area in the brain in which smell and taste are recognized.

In around a third of people the sense of taste and smell will return; if it has not come back in six months or so, it is unlikely to do so.

Loss of the sense of smell can be a serious handicap. Apart from the pleasures of food and wine, smell is an important safety sense, warning us of fire and escaping toxic substances such as petrol and gas. People working with solvents, paints, and plastics are at particular risk. People who have lost their sense of smell must be warned and told how to avoid exposure to danger. The occupational therapist will help them to carry out household tasks, such as using timers to warn them when food will have cooked rather than depending on the smell.

Even though they have not actually lost the sense of smell, after a head injury some people may complain that food tastes different. They may no longer like some foods or develop an appetite for things they never touched before. This is probably due to some damage to the brain itself rather than to the nerves of smell.

Sight

In a serious injury sight can be damaged in a number of ways. The ability to see can be lost by an injury to the eye itself or the nerve which connects it to the brain. Seeing to one side may be impaired, as we mentioned above. A commoner problem is interference with the way that the eyes follow and focus on a target. They need to swivel in their sockets so that each is pointing exactly to the target, with an adjustment so that they converge when it is closer. At the same time the lens of the eye has to alter so that the image is focused, and the pupil of the eye adjusts to the amount of light available. Injury to any of the several nerves concerned or to the complex central mechanism in the brain that controls them will result in blurred or double vision.

Even before consciousness returns it may be obvious that something is wrong, perhaps because one pupil is dilated or one eye skewed. Until they are fully awake the patient may not notice the problem, as the disordered sight from the affected eye may be suppressed. When they begin to notice the problem and complain, it will be best to put a shade over one eye, cutting out the confusing image. In the early days no other treatment is needed, and usually there is considerable improvement and sometimes complete recovery over the next few months. When it seems that no more recovery can occur, the alignment of the eyes can often be improved by an operation on the eye muscles.

Sometimes the main complaint is loss of sharpness of vision; older people need new glasses and younger people who have had no problems before may find that they need spectacles to see clearly. In many cases this is because before the accident they were having to compensate for impaired vision by continual effort from the mechanisms in the brain which adjust the focus and alignment of the eyes. After the head injury this effort is too great, the adjustment doesn't occur and vision is blurred. Again, improvement often occurs over a period of months and it may be wise not to make expensive adjustments to glasses without giving time for vision to improve.

Another troublesome symptom is intolerance of bright light, known as photophobia. This again wears off in time, and until it does it is best to use dark glasses, especially when out of doors.

Body temperature

In Chapter 2 we explained how the brain stem is the part of the brain that is responsible for body functions that we do not control consciously. Body temperature is one of these functions. When the brain stem has been damaged, temperature control can be less efficient. Sometimes people feel abnormally cold, even in the middle of summer. They may need to use electric blankets or heaters when people around them are complaining of the heat, and pile on extra clothes when everyone else is down to the minimum. In most cases this sensation of excessive cold is part of the way that the body signals that it is tired. Normal temperature control often returns when they are no longer fatigued.

Altered temperature control can also be shown by feelings of excessive heat, with the same problems as those noted in the last paragraph. Again, it seems to be linked to fatigue, and the extent of the problem varies with the degree of tiredness. Apart from the fact that they may attract some odd looks because their clothing is not normal for the season, this problem with temperature control is not life threatening, or something that you need to worry about. Let them determine the clothing and environment that they need to be comfortable.

Stress

We all understand what it means to experience stress. Stress occurs when we are put under pressure, in a way that tests our ability to cope. Typically, our body reacts to sudden physical or mental challenge in a number of different ways. Heart rate speeds up, there is a rush of adrenalin and breathing becomes more rapid and shallow. At the same time blood vessels in the gut and skin suddenly narrow, making more blood available to the muscles. Hence the expression 'white as a sheet'. All of these changes add up to the 'stress response', the body's way of preparing for 'fight' (face the challenge), or 'flight' (escape from danger). A mild stress response may produce 'butterflies' in the tummy, while a more extreme reaction may lead to feelings of heightened anxiety, fear, or panic. The capacity to react quickly to threat or danger is a useful human trait. A moderate level of anxiety can help us meet a deadline, achieve a goal or remain alert when it is important to do so. It is normal to respond to stress by becoming more energized for a time. This can be very effective in helping us cope with a crisis or challenge.

Thus we can see that the healthy stress response involves changes in our body, changes in our feelings, and often changes in our thinking as well. All three aspects, sensation, emotion, and thinking can be altered by a head injury. Deficits of perception, insight, and judgement may affect the way that the world is experienced, so that things we would consider stressful, such as trying to cross a busy motorway on foot, may not worry the person recovering from a head injury. On the other hand things that we take for granted, such as the ability to screen out background noise, and bustle, may be very stressful for the person recovering from the head injury.

However, there is another kind of stress which does not involve the 'fight or flight' response. This is the stress which results from situations or events which are not temporary, but which are part of our normal lifestyle. Some parents do have to cope with the behaviour of a delin-quent teenager, some partners do need to continue living with an alcoholic, most people do learn to manage the stress and pressure of remaining within a budget. However, after a head injury it is not unusual for the ability to cope with this kind of stress to be affected. Problem solving and decision making will be hard for a while, as we explained in the last chapter, and fatigue is a major factor in limiting how much head-injured people can handle. They cannot always quickly deal with situations as they had done before the accident, and the stress of this change compounds their normal lifestyle stress. The sleep pattern can be disturbed, so that fatigue becomes more of a problem, headaches develop and their ability to function reduces even more.

It is important that your family member or friend seeks advice and help if they are in this situation. They need counselling and some help with stress management, and also often benefit from using whatever relaxation technique suits them best. It is important that they under-stand that there are many different relaxation techniques, so if one does not help them to relax, the therapist needs to be told so that he or she can try them with another method. Sometimes practical inter-vention may also be needed. For example, if they are stressed by the impossibility of stretching an income that is reduced because they are no longer working, budget advice and approaches to banks and mortgage holders on their behalf to arrange extended time for repayment will certainly help.

Post-traumatic stress disorder

Another debilitating, but much less common, stress disorder can affect people who have been exposed to situations of extreme threat, danger or fright. Awareness of Post-Traumatic Stress Disorder (PTSD) has grown in recent years and most of us know that wars and other disasters can bring on stress problems that continue to plague the sufferer long after the original crisis has passed. Diagnosis of PTSD is complex, but the most characteristic symptom is the presence of intrusive thoughts or 'flashbacks' of the incident that are often associated with vivid sensations and powerful feelings of panic.

On the face of it, one would think that people who have been in a head-injury accident must run a high risk of developing PTSD. However, the evidence shows that the reverse is true, and that this kind of stress reaction happens less often than might be expected from comparison with the effects of major disasters or torture. As yet there is no agreement as to why this should be, but it is reasonable to suppose that the memory loss associated with closed head injury serves a protective function. If you cannot remember the accident that caused your injury, you cannot be troubled by nightmares and panic reactions about it. However, if you do have reason to suspect that you or someone you care for may be suffering from undiagnosed PTSD in addition to the effects of head injury then you should speak to the rehabilitation team, or to your family doctor. Bear in mind, though, that this is a rare situation, and perhaps no more than two or three percent of persons who have had a head injury will have PTSD as well.

Case histories

Samuel

Six weeks after his fall Samuel came home from his grandparents. His parents and older brothers welcomed him back with his favourite takeaways, and almost every person in his school football team called to see him. It was a very exciting time for everyone, and Samuel talked with his friends about being back at school the next week, after yet another orthopaedic appointment to X-ray his leg. By early evening he began to flag a little, and had the first headache he had experienced since the first few days at the coast.

Suddenly he stopped talking in the middle of a sentence and stared vacantly into space, then he said something that sounded like a word, but which didn't mean anything, over and over again. After what seemed like ages, but was only a few minutes, he blinked and then began to cry, saying he had a headache. He was put to bed and slept right through the night. Next morning he did not remember anything of the incident. The family doctor was called, and after he had talked with Samuel and the other members of the family he arranged an appointment with a neurologist.

While he was waiting for this Samuel returned to stay with his grandparents, even though the orthopaedic specialist was very pleased with how well the fracture was healing, and had said that he could start doing some gentle exercise at school! By the time he saw the neurologist he had had no more funny 'turns', and when an EEG turned out to be quite normal for boys of his age it was decided that he could safely return home and start back at school, especially as there was only one more week before the vacations started.

Jonas

Jonas settled down into a routine after the angry outburst which had ended up in the police station. He spent each morning in the occupational therapy department, at first in the woodwork and technical room, but this part of the programme was soon modified. Although he was almost out of his apprenticeship as a carpenter he could not work from a plan, found it impossible to figure out which part of an assembly fitted where, and could not manage tasks which needed two hands, such as threading a nut on a bolt. Not only was his left hand clumsy and would not go where he wanted it, but he could not judge with his eyes how far apart the pieces in each hand were.

After a week of this Jonas was prepared to work on the problem. His occupational therapist and Stephen and Suzy talked with him about setting up a programme with more realistic goals. These goals were not the ones Jonas had set when he had left the head-injury ward. At that stage his aims had been to get back to work and to move back to living independently of his parents.

Now he realized that he needed to learn how to make his hands work together, and to learn how to 'see' things properly again, and to be able to make sense of maps and plans and diagrams. He no longer needed to be bribed by the prospect of learning to look after himself in a flat. He had realized that there were things that had been affected by the accident, and thus he took the first steps towards his acceptance of the importance of rehabilitation.

Pauline

Pauline was doubly disadvantaged by the accident. She was disadvantaged as a person on the brink of middle age, and she was disadvantaged as a professional person who had a very demanding job. She was very aware that she was not well enough to return to work, but was not sure why. She could not think clearly, and felt as if she was in a dream and detached from the world around her. Each visit from friends or colleagues ended either with her in tears or with a massive migraine-like headache. Her husband John was convinced that she had developed a post-traumatic stress disorder, and read all he could about this in the library at the local medical school. Unfortunately he did not also read up on the effects of closed head injury, and saw her tiredness, emotionality and 'reluctance to return to work' as evidence that he was right in his diagnosis. He determined to help her recover from this, and to this end set up tasks to get through each day. He worked out a schedule for her which did not allow her time to sit and fret about the accident, and which he thought would take her out of herself.

The results were exactly the opposite, and Pauline became worse instead of better. She could not complete even half of the tasks, could not cope with even one visitor a day, let alone the cheer-up groups that John had organized, and became more and more uncoordinated as the days wore on. She had continual disabling headaches, and by the end of the second week began to have trouble getting to sleep at night, and trouble staying asleep. Eventually a worried colleague persuaded John to take her to see his family doctor.

To John's surprise he did not question Pauline about how stressed she felt by the accident, or ask her about 'flashbacks' or panic attacks. Instead he asked about her memory of the event, and how well she could concentrate. He explained to them both that her disordered sleep pattern was because she was not allowing herself time to recover and was getting over-tired. He asked how she was spending her day, and when John described the daily schedules that he had set up for her his only response was to comment that it made him feel exhausted to hear about it!

He explained to them both that even someone in their twenties needs two or three weeks to recover from an injury such as hers, and that some of them need much longer. He pointed out that as people age they take longer to bounce back, and that Pauline needed to expect that it might take at least three months and not weeks, since she needed to be more robust to return to work than if she had a less demanding occupation. While they were still with him he set up arrangements for her to attend an out-patient rehabilitation programme that had been specially set up for people with less severe head injury problems.

The first week on this programme was spent learning tricks to help her relax, and working through different techniques until she found one that worked for her. She learned to recognize signs of stress and fatigue, and slipped into a routine of short periods of productive activity with long periods of restful sleep in between. By the end of the second week even John noticed the improvement. He found that he looked forward to collecting her from the rehabilitation centre after work, and the family evening meal times again became the nicest part of the day.

7 Needs of particular groups

Statistics show us that more than 50 per cent of all head-injury cases are young men aged between 17 and 25 years and that most of the injuries happen in road traffic accidents. The two next largest groups are pre-school children who fall from windows, down stairs, or from playground equipment, and old people who are mostly injured in falls at home. People in these and other special groups can all have the same sorts of problems that were discussed in Chapter 5, but often with important individual variations. This chapter discusses the particular problems that head injury raises for some special categories of people and what can be done to help them. However, remember when you are reading this section that all cases are different. Not all small children will have the problems that we talk about and not all older people will find head injury so difficult to overcome.

The head-injured small child

Small children have special problems after head injury for several reasons. The first is the difficulty which they have in understanding what has happened to them and in passing on how they feel to their parents. It is unlikely for example, that their vocabulary will include the words 'headache' or 'dizzy'.

Adults who have had a head injury often have difficulty with self control and they may express this with physical aggression. A child is only just beginning to learn self-control, so it is not surprising that tantrums are common after the accident, and that injury to self and to others can occur. Parents will notice that the child's behaviour is worse when he is tired, and they need to make sure that he has plenty of rest. They should watch the child carefully, and as soon as he shows signs of irritability he should be put to bed for an extra sleep. Other strategies which can help are to make sure that there are plenty of different activities available to keep the child's interest, and to give him a chance to work off his irritability with physical exertion, such as bouncing on a trampoline.

Parents may find that caring for a head-injured small child involves almost 24-hour supervision, and this is too much to expect from any person. If the problem lasts for any length of time then the parents need to make sure that there are relatives or friends who can help, to give them some time for themselves and for the other children.

The next reason why head injury at this age is a special problem is that the pre-school years are the time when a tremendous amount of learning takes place. By the time children are three or four years old they have not only acquired the basic skills of walking and manipulating the environment with their hands, but they can express simple concepts in speech, recognize what they see, and make simple comparisons. All of this depends on an effective memory but, as we have seen, this ability is very likely to be damaged in a head injury.

What does this mean for the child? Fortunately, the skills that he has already mastered are likely to be retained, although he may have some difficulty in using them because of other factors such as fatigue and irritability. From the time of the accident, however, the child may have greater difficulty in building on those skills, and he may progress more slowly than his peers. This is a cumulative process. If the accident occurred at a time when the child would normally be acquiring the ability to tell the difference between various shapes and angles, he will then find it difficult to tell the difference between letters making up a word. If the child then has difficulty in learning to read, he will fail in the next step of education, and so on.

Small children
May not be able to explain how they feel
May not be able to control irritability
May be restless and aggressive
May not learn well
May fall behind their peers

There is now some evidence that even an apparently trivial head injury during the pre-school years can affect the child's ability once he starts school. This may not be the case with your child, but if he does not seem to be keeping up with his classmates, it would be sensible to speak to the teacher about the fall or other accident that he had.

What can you do to help? A clue comes from what happens when head injury or some other condition damages the part of the brain that controls talking and language. Although to begin with speech may be lost completely, most children manage to understand speech and talk again quite quickly. Partly this is because the brain of the small child is not as 'specialized' as that of an adult, and it seems to be easier for other areas of the brain to take over the control of speech. Another reason why speech is regained may be that the child gets plenty of practice listening to words after he has had an accident. Parents and friends amuse the child with stories as special treats because he has just come home from hospital. Further, he has plenty of practice listening to family members talking between themselves. We have seen that constant repetition is the basis of rehabilitation techniques, and it may be that the constant exposure to speech which a child who has been in hospital is subjected to is a kind of informal rehabilitation procedure. It is possible that children may be taught in the same way, by constant repetition, to regain other skills which they have lost. Many children's games and activities are good practice for visual and perceptual abilities. Ask your child's pre-school teacher or occupational therapist to suggest puzzles which may help.

The head-injured schoolchild

Although the older child will already have established the language and visual skills needed to read and write, impaired memory will still be a handicap because the school years are obviously a period when the ability to learn is important. We know that the child might have problems with new subjects, such as learning a second language, and it is sensible to delay French lessons, for example, until memory is a little better. We also know that often a child who has had a severe head injury cannot remember some of the schooling that he has already done (this is because of the 'retrograde amnesia' described in Chapter 5). It is unfair to expect children to learn a particular level of mathematics if they have no memory for the previous time at school when the basics which are needed to cope with that level were covered. In this case it is sensible to put off the higher mathematics lessons, and to go over the learning that has been 'lost'.

It is not just the learning difficulty that a child may have after head injury which is a problem for them. The typical classroom with one teacher to up to thirty or so children is not an easy environment for any child to cope with after a head injury. A head-injured child will have concentration problems, so he will find it hard to keep his attention on the lesson and to ignore the many distractions in the room. He will probably take longer to do things, so he will not be able to finish his work in the same time as the other children. He will tire more quickly, and as he gets tired his concentration will deteriorate even further, and he is likely to become restless and labelled as having 'behaviour problems'.

It is easy to see how the child can be seen by his classmates and his teachers as naughty and/or stupid, even though before his accident his behaviour and achievement level may have been average or better. It is an unfortunate fact that children can be blunt and unkind in their reactions to others who are different in some way, and it often is impossible for the head-injured child to live down a 'dummy' label given at this stage. The issue of managing return to school after head injury is covered more fully in Chapter 9. Here it is important to remember that the need for the child to have contact with his peers has to be balanced against the importance of making sure that he has recovered sufficiently to cope with the experience without having his self-confidence destroyed.

Parents and care-givers are sometimes better able to estimate the staying power of their child and how much should be expected of him than are the rehabilitation staff, who may only work with the child for a few hours each week. However, as well as this information about how much the child can do before he tires, we also need to know how good his memory is, how fast his reaction times are, and how well he can concentrate, before we can reach a sensible decision about starting back at school. This is the sort of information that we can get from a good objective assessment carried out by an experienced rehabilitation specialist. This information will be used in guiding the return to school, and it is important to stress that this will not be started before the child is ready. Neither will it be delayed after he has regained sufficient ability to cope.

What about the child who was already having problems at school before the accident? Well, we can be very sure that the head injury is not going to make these problems any better. It is less easy to decide whether or not school is going to be even harder for the child. If the head injury was very severe your doctor will be more definite about the need to expect problems than if it was relatively minor. But in either case do make sure that you get advice about the process of returning to school. It also helps if the child can return to a school that is familiar to him, and to teachers who have taught him before.

We have talked mainly about the problems the older schoolchild has with learning, and with getting back into the school system. There are other problems. Time does not stand still, and as the months and then years since the accident slip past, younger brothers and sisters continue to grow and develop, and often overtake the head-injured child in social skills as well as in education. However secure and well adjusted he may seem to be, the teenage victim of a head injury will find it hard to be happy about a younger sibling starting to date before him, or succeeding on the sports field where he never could. Counselling, to help your child come to grips with the effects of the accident, may have been offered earlier on. Sometimes it is important to have counselling at a later stage also, and the child often is more receptive when events, such as seeing a younger brother do the things that they cannot do, bring home the reality of the accident to them.

There is indeed a good case to be made for counselling, or at least advice, to be given every six months or so to family, to friends, and to teachers. In the early stages after the injury no one needs reminding about the accident or the way it has affected the patient. As time goes by it is sometimes less obvious that the child has been injured and that he still has problems. Indeed there may be overt comments like 'But the accident was years ago, he must be recovered by now' when it is suggested that the schoolchild still cannot cope with a normal daily programme. As we point out in the next chapter, families often expect recovery to follow the same sort of pattern in everyone, and find it difficult to cope with the concept that the degree of recovery and the time it takes is uncertain. Regular counselling would also help parents to cope with the problems which may develop as their child grows into adolescence with a disability.

The head-injured elderly person

By the time people reach their sixth or seventh decade they will probably have found that they are more forgetful, a bit slower, and perhaps not quite as efficient as when they were younger. Certainly they will know that in matters of judgement and 'wisdom' they are in their prime, but they would probably hesitate to challenge a younger person to a competition which required making quick decisions. This is an inevitable, and normal, part of ageing. So already, even before the accident, the elderly head-injured victim has probably experienced some of the after-effects of a head injury to some degree. Thus it is not surprising that an older person usually is more incapacitated, and does not recover as quickly, or as completely, as someone in their teens or twenties. Yet the person is at an age when his years of experience often mean that he is at the peak of his career.

There are advantages and disadvantages to having an important position at work. The head-injured person may insist that he cannot take time off work because he is needed to run the ship, as it were. Or he may worry that he will lose his position of authority to his juniors if he is away too long. So he runs a real risk of returning to work before he has recovered well enough to cope with the work, and of failing. This puts a tremendous strain on the family, who find themselves in the position of having to tell father or mother that he or she is not good enough any more to handle the jobs which he or she have maybe done for a quarter of a century. And if, as so often happens, the elderly person does not have much insight into the head-injury problems, the family also have the task of correcting errors and picking up the pieces.

If your head-injured relative or friend falls into this age group, you will know by now that you can need as much help and support as he does. Pride may make it hard for you to let friends, or even other family members, realize how much he has changed. Pride may also make it hard for you to ask for help. If professional counselling is available then take advantage of it. In these cases it is usually easier to unburden your fears to an outsider.

We said that the fact that the elderly person has reached the peak of his career also has its advantages. One advantage is that he has no doubt learned some ways of compensating for the decline in memory that has crept up over the years. He has already learnt that he has to use the diary, the calendar, and the other memory aids which we talked about in Chapter 5. The other advantage is that often he is in a position to reorganize his role to that of adviser or mentor, and often can restrict the hours of work to those he can manage. Provided he is aware of the limitations that he has, he can modify his lifestyle so that the demands he makes of himself fall within his capacity at that stage.

It may be, however, that the best option is to take early retirement, and to use these extra years to develop a hobby or activity that there was never enough time for up until now. It is often more realistic to accept that the years of paid employment are over than to struggle to achieve the goal of 'return to work' when this is simply going to lead to frustration and disappointment. Your support as the carer will be very important at this stage, and you also will need to accept that this is a positive step which will make your own life, and that of the head-injured person, much less difficult.

> After head injury an elderly person is unlikely to recover as quickly or as completely as a younger person

So far we have concentrated on the elderly person who was still in the work force at the time of injury. People who have already retired may also have to make changes to their lifestyle, and these will often affect their independence. If your relative or friend lives alone and if memory and concentration problems put him at risk, for instance of burning his house down, it will be necessary to make arrangements for his safety. Your circumstances may be such that you can have your relative or friend to live with you, but you should remember that older people do not recover either as quickly or as completely as the young, and that the arrangement may turn out to be a permanent one.

The head-injured psychiatric patient

People with a history of psychiatric disorder can, like anyone else, suffer a head injury. If the person you are caring for comes into this category, it may be harder for him to deal with the head injury.

The general effects of the head injury may be very similar to those of his illness, such as tiredness, poor concentration, aggression, and mood changes. Because of his illness he may have less ability to deal with the more specific head-injury problems such as headache and dizziness or disabilities of movement, speech, and thought. Also, head-injury symptoms, such as the sleep disturbance that may occur, can make his psychiatric condition worse. Medication that a psychiatric patient needs may slow down his reaction times and affect his ability to concentrate, and the tests used to assess mental function after head injury may become misleading. It may therefore become very difficult to decide which condition is responsible for the symptoms he shows. Because you know him well, you may be able to do this better than the rehabilitation team, and thus be a great help to them. You can let them know the ways in which he has changed, and the things that were a problem to him even before the accident. You will also know the sorts of things that he responds to, and how *not* to treat him.

We have stressed the importance of support and counselling for carers and family members. You need to have the chance to talk with other people who have had relatives with similar problems. Sometimes this can be arranged through your local head-injury organization, and sometimes there will be someone in a psychiatric support group who can give you this help. In either case, while you have the task of caring for someone with both a disorder and an injury, you do need to use any agency that is available to provide a 'minder' for the patient, so that you can have some time to yourself and to spend with the other members of the family.

So far in this section we have talked about people who were suffering from a psychiatric illness when they had the accident. Unfortunately, there are also problems if the head-injured person has a history of such an illness some time in the past. Even though they may have been symptom-free for many years, or their symptoms have been well controlled by medications for years, their medical and other assessments can be coloured by this history. Further, the accident insurer may see the current problems as a recurrence of the illness, rather than as an effect of the accident. If this happens your friend or family member will need your help to overturn this decision. You will need to get statements from his employer and other people he associates with that verify your knowledge that he had been coping well until the time of the accident.

The head-injured substance abuser

A substance abuser has similar difficulties to the patient who has a history of psychiatric illness in that he has problems which existed before the head injury which often make it hard for the rehabilitation team to decide what effect the accident has had. In addition, if he has been taking drugs or alcohol for some time, he is likely to have had a damaged brain even before the injury, and as with the elderly patient, he is not likely to recover as quickly or as fully as someone who did not have this history.

A substance abuser is likely to have broken away from the family before the injury. In many cases, however, parents or spouses will still feel that they have a responsibility to be the care-giver, and will sometimes see the accident as a time to make a fresh start. Unfortunately this is usually doomed to disappointment.

While the head-injured person is still recovering from the accident, he will not be able to cope with the demands of a substance abuse programme. You will recall from Chapter 5 that at this stage concentration will probably be poor, the person is likely to be irritable, restless, aggressive, he will have difficulty coping with more than one person at a time, and so on. Equally importantly, he will probably have a poor memory and so will not remember what has happened from one session to the next. He may have poor self-control also, so that he cannot be expected to be responsible for his own behaviour. It is unrealistic to expect to get him off the habit now that you have him back. It is also unrealistic to expect that recovery will follow the typical pattern of other head-injured people. There are likely to be withdrawal symptoms and other unpleasant effects, and it is important that he has professional care during this stage.

Unfortunately, because of his lifestyle and the effects which his activities have on his ability, substance abusers are very likely to have falls, fights, and traffic accidents. It is equally unfortunate that, because of the special problems which the substance abuser has, he does not usually do well in rehabilitation. Again this is an area where you may need some professional counselling so that you come to terms with the fact that your help may not be enough to change him.

In terms of the number of people who have a head injury, the sub groups of children, the aged, the psychiatric or the substance-abuse patients, make up only about half of all cases. Most head-injury patients are young adult males. But again, although the head injury has the potential to damage the same basic physical or cognitive functions in each case, the way these affect the person can be different depending on their role.

The head-injured woman

Even in this last quarter of the twentieth century, in spite of feminism and equal opportunities, expectations of the sexes can be rather different. The 'Big boys don't cry, only girls cry' edict is by no means dead. If your head-injured friend or relative is a woman she is at risk of having genuine complaints of headache and fatigue treated more lightly than if she were a man. She may also find that emotional changes and weeping frequently can be ascribed to her sex rather than to the accident. Worse still, she may believe this herself, and think that she is going through a nervous breakdown. You can reassure her.

Men and women are different, but the effects of a head injury are present regardless of sex.

Many women also fill the traditional role of home-makers. Few societies recognize this as an occupation in the sense that paid employment is an occupation. Yet the job is probably more demanding and with worse working conditions than any other. What union would allow its members to work, or be on call, for 24 hours a day, seven days a week? What union would allow its members to carry out any number of unspecified tasks on demand; tasks as diverse as nursemaid, cook, gardener, and handyman. Homemakers accept this as part and parcel of bringing up a family, and families expect that the home-maker will be on call to do anything for them at practically any time.

What happens when the home-maker has had a head injury? You will have brought her home from hospital probably earlier than would have been the case if she had a 'proper' job waiting for her. She will find it difficult to accept that her role is now to be the cared-for rather than the care-giver. She may see the family doing her job rather incompetently, or at least in a different way from her own. She will also see that her children are not only sad and upset at her accident, but that they often have had to interrupt their schooling or careers to look after her. It is a complete role reversal for the family. Offspring have to comfort and guide the parent and partners have to assume the home-maker as well as the breadwinner role.

It is not surprising that she will resist attempts to get her to rest, and she will try to pick up the threads of her normal life again. In the early weeks after she comes home, while the accident is still fresh in your mind, you will find it easy to remember that she needs help. But as time goes by, especially if she looks as well as she did before the accident, it will be easy to slip into the expectation that she also will be able to cope as well as she did then.

The head-injured parent

We have talked about some ways in which a head injury affects the female patient. Obviously there are also role changes for any parent who has had a head injury. It is difficult for adult offspring to adapt to the change in role that this brings about. It is even more difficult if the offspring are still young.

Parents usually guide, criticize, and attempt to regulate the behaviour of their children. After a head injury, when their own behaviour may be socially inappropriate (for example, when they may laugh at the wrong time, or say what they think without worrying about the consequences), it is the children who have to do the monitoring. Younger children may be too embarrassed to bring their friends home after school, or fall into the habit of avoiding the head-injured parent because they do not know how to deal with the aggressive or irritating behaviour. Older children may also avoid coming home, or they may make the situation worse by over-reacting to what is seen as unwarranted attacks by the head-injured parent.

The uninjured parent is in the unenviable situation of attempting to act as referee, to hold the family together. However this parent reacts, either the children or the partner may feel that sides are being taken. It is very important not to let this type of adversarial situation develop. If it is your father who has a head injury, remember that he still sees his role *as* being a parent. You do not stop being his child just because of the accident. What you and your uninjured parent need to do is to build up a system where you can protect him from making costly or dangerous mistakes, but which allow him to maintain his dignity as an adult. He is not a child, so do not treat him as one.

It is tempting to think that family counselling will make things right. Family counselling should help you and the other parent cope with the situation, but it is unlikely to change the head-injured parent. He does not need to be counselled about his role as a parent. The problem is that he knows his role, but cannot, because of the accident, carry out the functions of a parent at this stage.

The head-injured partner

In a relationship where one partner has a head injury, it is the un-injured partner who carries most of the burden for keeping that relationship together. We have talked about role changes in this chapter. This is inevitable, because the effects of head injury prevent them from functioning in the way they did before the accident. Probably the most dramatic role change occurs where one member of a partnership has had a severe head injury.

Where the fit partner assumes the role of care-giver, the relationship becomes more akin to that of a parent and a child. The carer may still love the head-injured partner dearly, but as time goes by the responsibility for the care of the head-injured person can change this to a love which is more like that of a parent than a partner. This change will be fuelled by the inability of the injured partner to react in the same way as before the accident. Each time he or she is irritable, aggressive, or acts in an unreasonable way, their partner becomes more deeply entrenched in the role of a parent with the responsibility for correcting this behaviour.

Another barrier to the resumption of the old relationship is that sexual function is often disturbed after a head injury. In the early stages after discharge from hospital the head-injured person may tire too quickly to do anything but sleep when he gets to bed. There may also be physiological or hormonal changes which interfere with sexual activity. Even where the partnership was very sound, inability to have sexual relations puts a strain on both partners. The less robust partnership may well founder.

The person with a mild head injury

Paradoxical as it may seem, the person who has been unconscious for only a few minutes, and who was not badly injured enough to need to be admitted to hospital, may have as many problems as the severely injured person who did not regain consciousness for many weeks. This is because it is usually very obvious to those around him that the latter has been badly injured, and he is not expected to be able to do everything which he did before the accident as well as he did it then. A mildly-injured person, however, may have nothing to show that he has been injured, and so there is unlikely to be visible evidence that he has not recovered from this injury.

For the majority of these cases, this is only a temporary problem, and the head-injured person will get back his ability to concentrate, to remember, and to think quickly in just a few weeks. However, we know that 5–10 per cent will take much longer than that to recover, and that they can be disabled for many months. This slower than normal recovery is a special problem because people in this group have not usually spent more than a few hours in hospital and so they do not have access to rehabilitation programmes, even where these exist. In Chapter 4 we described how a follow-up appointment is usually given to a victim who has spent some time in hospital after a head injury, to check his progress, and we pointed out that this sort of system would be impractical for less severe injuries because of the sheer numbers involved.

There should be a system, however, where people who are likely to be at special risk after a mild head injury can be screened, and which can provide facilities for checking people who continue to have problems. For example, Accident Department personnel need to know that older people, as well as students and those who are in demanding jobs, should be referred for assessment of memory, concentration, and other problems that can follow closed head injury (see Chapter 5) before they get back to work or school. This assessment should be carried out two or three weeks after the accident, by which time the early unpleasant effects, such as nausea and sleeping all the time, should have passed.

Often, understanding the reason for the problems which he has, and a bit of advice about how to cope with them, is enough to carry the mildly-injured person through this stage. Some find that the opportunity to interact with other people who have the same problems is also useful. If your relative or friend is one of the number of people who is taking a while to recover after a minor head-injury then talk with your family doctor about referring them for this help.

Case histories

Samuel

Samuel's parents had already visited the school and spoken to his teacher. They told her about the turn that he had had, about the rules that the orthopaedic specialist had set about what Samuel should and should not do, and arranged for him to come home at lunch time so that he would not get too tired. They also arranged with Grandma that she come to stay for the first week so that someone would be with him in the afternoons.

The first morning at school started off well. The teacher had written a special 'Welcome back, Samuel' message on the blackboard, and all the other children were very nice to him. The first lesson was music, and Samuel was allowed to play the big drum, something everyone in the class looked forward to. Reading came next, and Samuel opened his book at the first page, but could make no sense of any of it, so just sat and pretended that he did. Then they had maths. While Samuel had been away the others had moved on to harder work, so the teacher gave him some revision exercises to do instead. He had never liked maths, but even the first easy sums on the page were like something in a foreign language to him. He was so frightened by this that he wanted to cry, but he was determined not to do so in front of the other children. He could not make sense of any of the numbers, and did the only thing he could think of to get them out of his sight; he carefully scribbled over each one so that it would disappear off the page.

Miss Jones had been moving around the classroom helping where people were stuck, and she glanced over at Samuel from time to time, and was pleased to see him concentrating so well on his work. By the time she reached his desk he had managed to cover up half the numbers. Miss Jones was so angry when she saw what he was doing that she sent him to stand at the front of the class. The other children began to whisper and giggle, which made Samuel so angry that he picked up the vase of flowers off Miss Jones' desk and smashed it on the floor. Then he stormed out of the room as quickly as his leg would allow him, hid himself in the cloakroom, and cried uncontrollably.

Later in the headmaster's office, with his mother looking stern, and also angry that she had been dragged away from her work, he tried to explain that he could not do the sums that he had been given to do. Miss Jones waved his work-book at him, and showed him that he had done the very same exercise the week before his accident, and had got almost half of them right. Very quickly the adults agreed that Samuel had become very spoiled and lazy since his accident, and was just trying to get out of work. They also agreed that he should be at school full-time once the vacation was over. The consensus was that if he had any more time off school he would never get back to doing any work again.

Even Grandma did not seem to understand when he told her about it that afternoon. She would not even let him watch television while he ate his lunch, and when he had finished, sent him off to bed. Almost immediately she heard a funny noise coming from his room. The noise came from Samuel. He was sitting on the floor with a very vacant look in his eyes and saying noises that sounded like words but were not, over and over. As he had done after the first turn, he started to cry after a few minutes, and complained again of a really bad headache. He fell asleep the minute his grandmother put him into bed, and was still asleep when the rest of the family arrived home from work.

Jonas

Jonas continued to make steady, though slow, progress and though he had not yet returned to the woodwork room he had learned to be more independent in daily living. Though he still had some problems getting his hands working together, especially when he was tired, and though he still found it hard to work out maps and diagrams, the rehabilitation team considered that he was ready to move to the next stage — living in a flat of his own. He had long since had to give up the flat he had shared before the accident, but there was supervised accommodation available in the grounds of the rehabilitation unit, and one of the flats was available for him.

Although his parents were a little apprehensive about how well he would cope, they looked forward to having their home to themselves again. There was another full family meeting with the team, and the accident insurer agreed to continue to employ Stephen for attendant care at the weekends. The occupational therapist arranged to work with Jonas in the flat in the mornings, to help him with meal planning and organizing his housework, and with budgeting. Afternoons would be taken up with the daily sleep period that he still needed, and with time in the physiotherapy pool.

Things went well until the first weekend. Jonas had gone with Stephen to see a movie in the afternoon, and on the way out of the theatre he ran into some friends from work. They insisted on taking them to the pub across the road for a drink and something to eat. Stephen was a little reluctant about this, as he had been given very strict instructions that there was to be no alcohol. At his insistence he and Jonas had fruit juice though the others had beer. There was much to-ing and fro-ing to the counter as the members of the little party chose their meals, and after a while Stephen realized that Jonas was getting rowdy and even more clumsy. He watched aghast as Jonas got up from his chair, took a step and crashed to the floor, obviously very intoxicated.

The friends were also alarmed, and sobered up very quickly as they helped Stephen get him back to the car. It was obvious that Jonas had been unable to resist the temptation of alcohol, and had persuaded one of his friends to share his beer with him. The friend was sure that at most he would have had only one glass, and was amazed that this would be enough to have such an effect. As they manoeuvred the rubber-legged Jonas into the car Stephen explained that people's ability to tolerate alcohol was usually affected after a head injury, and that was one of the reasons why alcohol was forbidden at this stage.

With the help of this now contrite and badly shocked friend Jonas was taken home and put to bed, and left to sleep it off. He woke the next morning with a massive hangover and vowed never to touch alcohol ever again. Stephen did not believe him, of course, and realized that he should not put temptation in his way as he had done that night.

Pauline

As Pauline learned to manage her fatigue better her time on the programme was cut back and she spent two full days at home instead. For the first time since she had completed her law degree when her youngest child was five, she was a full-time wife and mother again. She still needed to rest frequently, but she rather enjoyed 'playing house' as she called it to herself. She had been cleared to drive again, and was able to run the children to their after school activities and to take time to browse in the dress shops for clothes for herself and for them. The only thing she found she could not do was the supermarket shopping. Fortunately John had come with her the first time she had made the trip, and realized that after just a few minutes the noise, the crowd, the massive sensory input and the decision making was just too much for her, and he took her home before she collapsed.

After three weeks she started to feel guilty that she was not working, and began to wonder if she was really justified in leaving her work at the law firm to others, and to wonder how long it would be before they decided not to hold her job any longer. She talked about this with her counsellor at the rehabilitation centre, and the team there decided that she should have a follow-up assessment to check how close she was to being ready to start to think about work. John arranged a meeting for Pauline to talk with the partner she worked with, and the counsellor came with her. This was very helpful, as she was able to explain Pauline's progress to the partner, and to negotiate with him about a plan for her to do some work at home at her own pace to begin with, and to aim for part-time work when she did return to the office. The other advantage was that the counsellor was able to remind Pauline how supportive the partner had been at this meeting whenever she started to get stressed at how long it was taking her to get over the accident.

There were also other causes of stress. Pauline and John had been used to a very full social life, and had a wide circle of friends. After a few rather disastrous evenings they agreed that they would not accept any more invitations to dinner, and restrict their outings to lunches or brunches. The first invitation after Pauline was well enough to go out was to accompany two other couples to a restaurant they both enjoyed.

They had forgotten the live music, the crowded tables, and how all the diners had to shout at the top of their voices to be heard. Pauline left the table even before the waiter came for their order, and one of the other women found her retching and sobbing in the ladies' restroom. After this they accepted an invitation to a quiet dinner with no other guests. This went reasonably well to start with, but by nine o'clock Pauline could barely keep her eyes open, and John had to take her home even though dessert had not yet been served.

After this she began to see herself as a handicap for John, rather than the strong competent partner that she had been up to now, and they had their first serious argument for many years when she tried to talk with him about this and he accused her of imagining things.

8

How long will it take for the patient to recover?

If you break an arm or a leg in an accident your doctor can usually tell you, to within a few days, how long you will need to be in hospital, for how long you will need to wear a plaster cast, and often how long it will be before you will be able to go back to work. If you also received a head injury in that accident most of these predictions become invalid.

Perhaps the most common complaint that families of a head-injured person make about hospitals and hospital staff is that no one can give them a definite answer to questions such as 'Will the patient live or die?' or 'When will the patient get better?' We have already explained in Chapter 3 that this is because the real answer to these questions is often 'We do not know yet. We will have to wait and see'. Although there are sophisticated machines and procedures to monitor brain function, these are never able to give a definite answer about how well someone will recover from a severe head injury. Many of you will have been warned that there is a possibility that your relative or family member might die, or at least become a 'vegetable'. It should be a matter of delight when neither of these events occurs. Instead, a more favourable outcome is often taken as evidence that 'they do not really know anything about head injury'. The fact is that 'they' do, and all the information which was available at that stage showed that there was a possibility of a poor, or no, recovery.

Given that in the early stages after injury it is not always possible to be definite about whether a patient is going to live or die, it is not surprising that many other questions about recovery are also difficult to answer. This chapter looks at some of the most common 'when' and 'how' questions.

When will the patient wake up?

Two different ways are used to describe the stage where a patient is 'asleep' after a head injury. These are that they are 'in a coma' or that they are 'unconscious'. Both mean the same thing although the coma description is the more usual. We have described the ways that your friend or family member is constantly watched while he is in a coma and how there is sometimes regular monitoring of the electrical activity of the brain. As long as there are no changes in these recordings it will usually not be possible for your doctor to tell you how long it will be before the patient will wake up. When there are changes, you may hear the word 'lightening' used. This simply means that the patient is in a less deep coma. In other words, he has already started to react to more things around him. However, it still might take days or weeks for him to move out of the 'coma' stage.

Do not expect a patient to open his eyes, stretch out his arms, and say 'Where am I?' as patients often do in movies or books. People rarely move abruptly from being in a coma to being properly awake. When the patient first starts to take notice of things around him he is likely to be quite confused about where he is and why he is there. He is likely to ask you again and again what happened to him, or why you have not been to see him before, even though you may have spent almost every waking hour at the hospital for many weeks! At this stage he is starting to 'wake up' but he is still not able to remember things that happen to him, probably from one minute to the next. Do not be alarmed, therefore, if the reaction to you is the same again after you have left the room briefly, perhaps to check something with the nurse, or when you return to visit at the start of a new day. Neither should you be alarmed if he appears to have 'lost' several years of life and insists that he is still at school, for example. We described in Chapter 5 how the memory of things that happened both before and after the accident is always disturbed for a while when there is a closed head injury.

Like the stage where the person is unconscious, or in a coma, this stage in which he is confused, repeats himself, and forgets things might last for a short time only, or for days, weeks, or months. It is clear that he is not properly awake, and we compared it to sleepwalking in Chapter 5. So you see that to answer the question of when the patient will wake up, your doctor would need to be able to predict not only how long he will be unconscious, but also how long this confused stage will last. Thus there are two 'when' questions. However, when your relative or friend is past the coma stage, your doctor will have a better idea about how long the next stage will go on for. This is because the confused state usually lasts longer the longer the period of coma has been. This rule of thumb does not allow your doctor to give you the day and date when the patient will 'wake up'. The doctor can tell you things like 'He will probably be like this for a few months yet', or 'He will probably be more aware of things in a few days'; beyond this you simply have to accept the 'wait and see' advice.

These periods of changed consciousness are a time when you, even more than the hospital staff, can help your relative or friend wake up a bit more. You can tell them what music he liked, what his interests were, what he liked to be called. You can bring photos and mementoes in to the hospital ward to remind him of his real life. It is your voice that he will recognize and which is familiar to him, not the voices of the nurses and doctors. Also, you will probably spend more time with the patient each day than any one member of the hospital staff, so you can be an important observer to watch out for changes in the things that he can do.

The hospital staff may suggest to you that you keep a daily journal of this period. Not only will this give you something to do while you are waiting for the patient during the frequent naps that he will take, but also it will be a valuable record for the days and weeks ahead. It is only natural that there will be times when you feel very down and depressed about things, especially when you cannot see much progress from one day to the next. These are the times to get out your diary and remind yourself of how he was only a month or two back, and to realize how much improvement there has been since then. Your relative or friend will also appreciate your work because, as we explained in Chapter 5, he is unlikely to remember anything of the early weeks when he was in hospital. Later on, when he is able to, he will read about what you and he went through.

When will the patient walk and/or talk?

In Chapter 6 we described how some patients may be paralysed, or have problems with balance and walking for a while after the accident. Others may have trouble making themselves understood when they talk. Because every accident is different, and every person who has an accident is different from every other, it is usually impossible for the doctor or therapist who is looking after your relative or friend to answer these questions. They will be able to tell you about any progress, and will probably do this without being asked because they are also excited about improvement in the patients they are working with.

The problem for you is that while your relative or friend is in the 'Head-Injury Ward' you will have seen many other patients at different stages of recovery. You will have talked to their family members about their accidents and when they happened, how their family members were affected. They will have told you how long it was before they managed to do different things. Why is this a problem? It can be a problem if this leads you to expect that your relative will recover in the same time. It is tempting to assume that because somebody's son is the same age as yours, and has had the same sort of accident, they will start to walk again after the same number of weeks. There are many things which influence how quickly or how fully your relative will recover, including the way the brain was injured in the accident. Again you just have to wait and see, and take things one day at a time.

This does not mean that you should not talk with other families in the ward. It is very important that you do. Even your closest friends or relatives will not understand what you are going through as well as someone who is in the same situation as you are. Many wards will arrange for you to meet with other people who have had a head injury in the family, and many areas now have voluntary agencies which run support groups for families (Appendix B gives contact addresses for the UK, USA, and Australasia). The point we are making here, and it is something that the other people at the support groups will tell you also, is that you cannot use the recovery pattern and recovery times of any other patient to judge how long your own head-injured relative or friend will take to recover the same skills.

When will the patient leave hospital?

Even though you know that the answer to this question will probably be the same as to the others — that is, we need to wait and see — there are some instances when you need to have a more definite answer. One consequence of an extended period in hospital after a head injury is that the person has been removed from his normal home and family life, without having had any chance to prepare for such a prolonged absence from home and work. Yet, until he recovers full consciousness, he will not be able to cope with the effects of this absence.

Following the accident the family has to make many practical decisions for the head-injured person. Rent and mortgages continue to come due whether the home is occupied or not. Should you sublet the flat, give up the lease, sell the house, or put in tenants? Employers have a right to expect that their employees will arrive for work each day. Should you ask the employer to hold the job, to put in a temporary replacement for him, or to accept his resignation? To make these decisions you need to have some estimate about the length of time the person will be in hospital. Usually these issues arise when there has not been very much progress for some weeks after the accident. When you explain the problems to your doctor, he or she will usually be able to advise you, even if he or she cannot tell you exactly how long your relative will be in hospital.

The next most important staff member for you to talk to is the Social Worker. This person will know who to get in touch with in the community, either to put things on hold, or to help you make financial and other arrangements. If your relative is an adult you will find that most countries have quite stringent rules that must be followed before you can use his bank accounts, alter contracts that he has entered into, or sell his property for him. This legislation was developed to protect people from the unscrupulous, and although you may find it rather offensive that anyone could consider that you would not act in the best interest of the head-injured person, it is important to go through the necessary steps if he is likely to be in hospital for an extended period.

When will the patient be better?

The more time which has passed since the accident, the more information your doctor will have about the kind of injury which your relative has had, and the more the doctor will be able to tell you about how much better he is likely to get, or in less severe cases, when he is likely to have recovered. We have already seen that once the doctor knows how long the patient has been unconscious, he or she will be able to give you some idea about how long the period of confusion will last.

These two after-effects of the accident, coma and the period of confusion and disturbed memory, are used as one of the ways of describing how serious a head injury has been. Generally, the longer the person has been unconscious, and the deeper the stage of coma when he reaches the hospital after the accident, the more badly he has been hurt. Information about how long the 'sleepwalking' stage lasts also gives a clue to how serious the injury has been. Obviously, the worse the injury the longer the patient is going to take to recover, and the less complete this recovery is likely to be.

These two measures can only give an estimate, an educated guess, about recovery and recovery times in any one patient. It is true, in general, that someone who has been in a deep coma for six months will make a less complete recovery than someone who has been unconscious for an hour. But there are some individual cases who make a better or faster than predicted recovery, and others who do worse than expected.

We have stressed that prediction becomes more accurate the more time which has passed since the accident, and the more information there is about how much the patient can do. By the time the person leaves hospital he will have recovered the ability to breathe for himself, move about more or less on his own, and communicate with other people, even if his talking is a little slurred or hesitant. He will be able to dress and feed himself, and manage his own toilet. He may still be a long way from being completely recovered, however.

How information builds up about the injury
How deep is the coma?
How long does the coma last?
How long does the 'sleepwalking' last?
How many physical problems are there?
How well do attention and memory work?
How quickly are problems improving?

Chapter 5 describes some of the problems which the patient may have at this stage. These problems can give you some clues as to how quickly he will get better. If the ability to concentrate is very poor, for example, this will affect everything he does. He will not remember things very well because his attention wanders, he will not progress as well with out-patient therapy because he cannot keep his attention on what he should be doing, and he does not practise the exercises at home because he forgets about them. In short, if his concentration is still very poor when he leaves hospital then he will take longer to recover than someone whose concentration is only mildly affected.

One of the important things about being able to answer the 'When will the patient be better?' question is to know how many of the after-effects of head injury the patient has, and how severe these effects are.

Then, of course, your doctor will need to know how quickly these after-effects are improving. This is why your relative or friend will be tested quite often after he has left hospital. Knowing how quickly he is improving will allow your doctor to give you some idea of when your relative will be better, but again it will only be an informed guess.

There are many other things apart from how serious the injury was which influence how quickly the patient will recover. One of the most important is further damage to the brain. This might happen if the patient injures his head again in another accident, or if he uses alcohol or other drugs which have an effect on the brain. It will obviously take longer to recover from one accident if the brain is continuously being injured.

Another factor which affects how quickly the person will recover is what he does while he is waiting to 'get better'. We know that people who have had a head injury are often not able to cope with stress very well, and if your friend or relative is worried about things — his job, money, relationships, or his own health — he will most likely not be able to relax, or to get enough sleep, and sometimes he may appear to be getting worse. It is important that you talk with your doctor about this, because this situation often can be helped with stress management programmes or with mild relaxants.

As you might expect, how quickly a patient will get better also depends on what kind of rehabilitation is available for him. We know that he will get better faster if he can get into a head-injury facility where he can be given a fully structured programme, alternating activities and rest according to his needs, and which will provide an environment where he is not likely to do further injury to the brain, or to develop stress reactions. In other words, there are suitable conditions where recovery is more likely to take place, and to take place more rapidly.

Recovery depends on
The severity of the injury
Whether there is further brain damage
Minimizing stress
Effective rehabilitation
Management of return to work/school

This section has dealt mainly with people who will make a fairly good recovery eventually. They are the people who can be expected to return to work or to school. How this is managed also affects how well and how quickly they will recover. In the next chapter you will find suggestions to help make the move back into the workplace or school as smooth and trouble-free as possible. Finally, there are some people, such as the elderly, who are less likely to make a speedy recovery. These special groups were discussed in Chapter 7.

We have seen that there are several things, apart from the injury, that determine how quickly your friend or relative will get better. To some extent these factors are also important in answering the next question, which is about those people who are unlikely to ever make a full recovery.

How much recovery can be expected?

Almost without exception you can be sure that your relative or friend will be better, sometime in the future, than he is today. How much better he will be is another matter.

We do not expect people who have lost a limb in an accident to grow another one. We know that the disability is permanent, even though a very good artificial limb might be fitted to help compensate for the missing one. With this sort of aid, a person is able to do most of the things that he could before the injury. Brains are different. Although we know that a person who has damaged parts of his brain will never regenerate them, we do not have any replacement for these areas. Yet in spite of this, we know that the patient can quite often get to do some of the things that a particular bit of the brain controlled. How can this happen?

Sometimes it is because the bit of the brain which is needed to allow the patient to do the activity was not destroyed, but could not work properly for a while because of swelling and bruising. Or it may have been that another bit of the brain which was needed to work with the control part was out of action for a while, for the same sort of reasons.

This kind of 'recovery of function', or getting back an ability which was affected by the head injury, generally takes place in the earlier period after the accident, and it generally happens whether or not you are trying to practise that skill.

Sometimes recovery happens because parts of the brain which are not damaged get used to taking over some of the job of the damaged bit. How this happens we do not know exactly, but it is clear that if the brain is to find a new way to do the particular activity which has been damaged, that activity has to be practised many times.

There are two important points about recovery after brain damage. The first is that how soon and how much improvement takes place is affected by the frequency and type of rehabilitation. The other important point is that there is always a limit to how much recovery can take place. This limit is set by the kind of injury, the amount of damage, and the age and lifestyle of the head-injured person.

The two-year myth

Many older textbooks make a very clear but quite incorrect statement about recovery after a head injury. They say that all the recovery that can be expected will take place in the first two years after the accident. This is simply not true. Not only is it not true, but it has caused much needless stress and unhappiness in families and patients who were given this incorrect information. You do not need to retire to bed on the eve of the second anniversary of the accident, believing that if your relative or friend is not walking yet, for example, then he is doomed to spend the rest of his life in a wheelchair. This may indeed be so, but two years is much too soon after the injury to give up hope, and to give up trying.

> People have continued to improve five, ten, or more years after a head injury

It is correct that the time when the most recovery takes place is in the first six months after the injury. This is partly because of the mechanism we described earlier where parts of the brain cannot work properly in the early stages because of bruising and swelling around them. But because improvement takes place at a slower rate in the next six months does not mean that it will eventually slow to zero.

If you are given the two-year myth, ask your doctor to confirm what we have told you. You might also like to ask around at the next Head-Injury Support Group which you attend. You will find no shortage of people to tell you about the progress which their relatives made well beyond the two-year period.

Support for the care-giver

You will see from the last section that when we talk about recovery after a head injury we are talking about what can be a very long-term affair. Even if your relative or friend eventually regains his independence, he may need you as a care-giver for many months. You will need to support him when he feels despondent about how little progress he has made. You will need to comfort him if his old friends neglect him, or if his brothers or sisters no longer bring their friends home to visit.

There are two things that you need to do. The first is to bring out that diary which we talked about earlier, the one you started while he was still in hospital. Read it through with him and you will be amazed at how much progress there has been since then. You will, we hope, have kept up with making a daily entry in this diary. The second thing which you need to do is to compare how the head-injured person is now with how he was two or three months ago, not with how he was before the accident happened.

Chapter 10 talks about coping with the long-term adjustments which need to be made when someone in the family has had a severe head-injury, and will never make a full recovery. Use some of that advice to get you through the stage when you are helping your relative or friend on the road to an independent life. We have already given you the most important advice, however, which is to look forwards and not back. Make the comparison between how he is now and how he was a few months ago, and set some realistic goals about how you would like him to be in a few months' time again.

Finally, you need to realize that you will not be able to help anyone if you make yourself ill looking after him. Allow yourself to have days off. Even if you do not have any relatives or friends who can mind the patient for you, the social worker at the hospital, or else your Head-Injury Society Support Group, will arrange for someone to sit with him. Do not be shy about asking for this help. Further on down the track you will be able to do the same thing for another family, and you will find out just how rewarding it is to give another carer a break.

Case histories

Samuel

The family doctor made an urgent appointment for Samuel to see the neurologist again after the second seizure. Samuel's mother and grandmother were devastated that they had been so ready to ignore his own account of his first day back at school. They realized that they had been so pleased to hear that the EEG results were normal that they had not wanted to take in the family doctor's warning that this did not necessarily mean that Samuel did not have 'post-traumatic epilepsy'.

The neurologist arranged for Samuel to be admitted to hospital for observation and monitoring, before starting him on anti-convulsant medication. He listened carefully while Samuel described how he could not make sense of things that were written on paper. He also listened carefully to the descriptions of Samuel's seizures, and explained that while the lad was in hospital he would have some memory and other tests to make sure that his treatment and rehabilitation would be appropriate. And so Samuel ended up spending the first few days of his school holidays in a hospital bed. One of the good things about it was that his teacher, Miss Jones, was his very first visitor, and she brought him a large toy goose with a label round its neck reading: 'MY NAME IS MISS JONES. I AM A SILLY GOOSE'.

Two of Samuel's older brothers were home when he came out of hospital, because it was also vacation time at the technical institute that they attended. They made sure he took the anti-convulsant pills that the neurologist had given him, and at the right time. They also took him to the zoo and the park and the movies, and waited at home with him for a new participant in his rehabilitation to call. This was his case manager from a paediatric rehabilitation service. She explained that because the neurologist had said that Samuel needed to be stabilized on his anti-convulsants before he started back at school, he would have lessons at home at first.

Samuel also had a visit from the tutor who was going to work with him. He talked about the results of the neuropsychological assessment that had been done in hospital, and left a bundle of games and puzzles that his brothers could help him with. Slowly the panic that Samuel had been living with since that awful morning when he first went back to school began to fade, and he realized that people did understand him and did want to help him.

Jonas

As Jonas gradually learned to look after himself in his 'supervised living' accommodation, the rehabilitation team's label for the unit he was renting, he became more anxious to take the next step in his independence, to be cleared to drive a car again. He had no memory at all of the evening of the accident, and although Stephen reminded him every time he brought the subject up that he had been charged with driving dangerously while above the legal alcohol limit, and was likely to lose his driving licence when the case came to court, this did not seem a real issue to him. The real barrier to him was that his car had been so badly damaged in the accident that it could not be driven and because he had not had any insurance cover he could not afford to get it repaired.

Stephen asked Suzy to arrange a family meeting to discuss Jonas's plan to work on the car himself. Both the neuropsychologist and the occupational therapist were concerned that he no longer had the skills he needed to see what the trouble was, or to get his hands working effectively to fix it. The social worker was concerned that if the car ever did get to a stage where it was roadworthy it would be difficult to enforce the ban on Jonas driving it. His parents were worried that if he did drive he would hurt someone else if not himself.

Eventually it was decided to set up a system to monitor carefully every step of the process as a practical vocational experience. His parents arranged for the car to be transported to a clear area near Jonas's unit. Suzy found a mechanic who was prepared to work with the occupational therapist to break down what was needed into small units, and who agreed to mark the work as either good, adequate or unsatisfactory as it was done. Stephen was to act as the 'job coach', monitoring what Jonas did at each stage. The accident insurer's representative agreed to fund the programme, but put a three month time limit on this.

This time limit was not needed. Before the end of the first month the team realized that the project was making Jonas worse rather than better. He was frustrated and angry that he could not manage simple repairs that he had done hundreds of times before. He could not understand why he no longer had the ability to replace a simple part without fumbling. His car had been his pride and joy, but although he knew what needed to be done he could no longer do it. After a particularly frustrating exercise with a spark plug he stormed off, and it took all Stephen's powers of persuasion to talk him into getting out of the taxi he had flagged down to take him to the nearest bar.

Pauline

John, Pauline's husband, was an intelligent and educated person. He had been very aware from the day of her accident of the changes that this had brought about. He could understand why these had occurred, but he could not understand why they could continue for so long. He did not talk about Pauline in the staffroom, but some of his colleagues did discuss their relationships, and before her accident he had been very aware how fortunate he was in his.

Now things were different, and he realized that it had been easier to cope in the early days after the accident, when it had been very obvious that she was not well. Now that she was so much better, and most of the time was back to the old Pauline, it was difficult to handle episodes of tears or irritability when these occurred. Although he knew that these only happened when she had spent too long working on the legal opinions that she was doing at home, he was not always able to resist an exasperated sigh or comment, which of course made the tears or anger even worse.

Pauline realized that her energy level, her ability to stay awake and alert, was still very limited, and that when she did test herself by cutting out the early afternoon sleep, John and the children suffered in the evening. She developed a routine of working for up to an hour in the morning, then pottering in the garden or listening to music for a while before getting back to another hour or so of her work. She had found that it was a total waste of time to try to do any more in the afternoons, even after she had had a sleep, so she kept that time for routine chores such as collating the morning's work.

Pauline was also concerned about her relationship, but when she attempted to talk things over with John he tended to change the subject, and focused on the children and some particular problem one of them might be having. Their social life continued to be very restricted, and for the first time since they had been married, Pauline did not accompany John to school functions, even when there was something that was held during the day. She held on to something her counsellor had said to her when she talked about how frustrated she was at not being able to do more. The advice was 'If you cannot have both quality and quantity, at least you have the quality'.

9 Back to work and study

For months everyone involved in the head-injured person's rehabilitation has been working towards getting him fit enough to go back to work, school, or college. Unfortunately return to work is sometimes botched, in spite of the very best of intentions. There are several ways in which this can happen. The person can be returned to work or school before he has recovered sufficiently to cope with it, often because neither the family nor the employer or school teacher want to hurt his feelings by telling him that it is too early. He can be returned to an inappropriate work or school environment because there has not been sufficient communication between the rehabilitation team, the employer or school, and the head-injured person and his family. Finally, things can go very wrong if there is no system for monitoring the success of the return to work or school trial. By looking at the ways in which return to work or school can go wrong, we can arrive at some general principles which we can use to set up a better system. Remember, however, that in this section we are talking about returning the head-injured person to the employment or study which he was doing at the time of the accident. This is not always possible.

After the description of an ideal 'back to work or school' system we discuss ways of finding an employment or educational slot that the person can cope with if the old slot is no longer the right one. The last part of the chapter talks about people with special employment problems; executives, the self-employed, the unemployed, the school dux, and the school dunce. Firstly, however, there are three basic questions about getting back into the real world.

Managing the return to work or school
Ensure that:
the head-injured person is well enough to go back
the head-injured person can cope with the environment
there is a system of monitoring the trial back to work or school

When is the head-injured person ready to go back to work?

There are quite clearly defined standards which head-injured people need to meet before they can be considered fit to work. The first is that attention and concentration span must be sufficient to allow them to work effectively and safely for a specified portion of the work day. The second is that they have maintained or regained the special skills that the job needs. The third is that they have the social skills which they need so that the return to work will not disrupt the routine of the workplace.

Before going back to work after a head injury
Attention and concentration must be adequate
The special skills required by the job must be adequate
Social skills must be adequate

From the time that the head-injured person wakes up after the accident and moves into the care of the rehabilitation team, the specialists will have been monitoring his ability to attend or concentrate, they will have been monitoring his ability to cope with the demands of the job or education, and they will have been monitoring his social skills. For this reason, the members of the rehabilitation team have all the information which is needed to answer the question about when return to work or study should begin. Problems arise if this advice is ignored.

Telling the head-injured person that he has not yet recovered sufficiently well to cope with work may not necessarily be enough to convince him that he is not yet ready. In Chapter 5 we explained how in the early stages after injury people often lack insight, and do not have the ability to judge how well they are doing. While he still has poor insight he will not be able to understand why he is being kept away from work, because it can seem to him that he does not have any problems. Sometimes even although he is aware that his memory is not as good as it used to be, or that he finds it difficult to concentrate, he may not appreciate that the way he copes with these problems makes it difficult for the other people at work or school. If he has to ask a question or pass on some information as soon as he thinks of it (because otherwise he will forget it), for example, or if he needs to get up and walk around or do something different when he cannot concentrate, employers or school teachers will not be impressed by the disruption which this causes.

If the person insists that he is right about fitness to work and that the rehabilitation team is wrong then it can be very difficult for the family. Even if the family have doubts themselves about whether or not the head-injured person will be able to cope, it can seem as if they are 'ganging up' against him if they try to persuade him to wait a while longer. It can also be difficult to resist the temptation to believe that perhaps he might be right after all. This is especially likely if families have had to listen to continual complaints that every activity which is suggested to him is boring, and that the only thing which he wants is to get back to work or to school. After a time families begin to doubt the explanation that the rehabilitation team gave that the 'boredom' is more likely to be frustration because the head-injured person does not have the ability to concentrate on the activities long enough to succeed, and because he tires so quickly that anything he does quickly becomes tedious. The family just want him to be happy.

Sometimes family members or friends do not understand how the head injury has caused the problems. They may label the person as lazy, unmotivated, or if they are teenagers, as 'anti-authority', 'anti-parent', or 'anti-school'. If this applies in your case, it is important that you arrange a meeting so that the relatives or friends can talk to the rehabilitation team. This will help everyone to understand why head-injured patients behave as they do, and if he is adolescent, which problems are to do with the injury and which are to do with growing up.

The situation becomes even more difficult if the employer or teacher also succumbs to the desire of the head-injured person to return to work or to school. In the typical scenario some time after the person has left hospital he calls to visit his employer. The employer may be unaware of the typical after-effects of head injury, or may not notice much change during the space of a short visit. If there are no obvious physical signs that he has not made a full recovery the employer is very likely either to ask him when he is coming back to work, or to agree to the suggestion that he starts back soon. On the other hand, where it is very obvious to the employer that the person is still impaired as a result of the accident, a misguided sense of compassion may lead him or her to offer to have them back at work whenever they want, and a promise that there will be something suitable for them to do.

In some cases the only practical way of managing is to allow them to have their way, and to find out for themselves. If they do go back to work too soon after a significant head injury they will soon find that the tiredness this brings on makes their other problems worse. They may complain of more frequent headaches, they may have more problems remembering things, and they may lose control of temper more often. The harder they try, the worse it may be. The tired, head-injured person makes more mistakes, forgets more messages, makes poorer decisions, and becomes more and more frustrated with the lack of progress which goes hand in hand with this sort of tiredness. If these problems are allowed to develop they can cause friction with other employees or with the employer. At best there may be a loss of job satisfaction, while at worst things may deteriorate and lead to demotion, redundancy, resignation, or dismissal.

Sometimes the decision about return to work is made without all the information from the rehabilitation team being used. This happens particularly when the family and employer are so impressed by the physical recovery that the head-injured patient has made that they assume that there has been equivalent recovery in cognitive function. It also happens when the accident has caused multiple injuries, and there are several different specialists involved. There may be a breakdown in communication between the different disciplines working with your relative or friend and the orthopaedic specialist, for example, may clear the victim as fit for work without being aware that he still has not recovered sufficiently from the head injury to cope. Unfortunately there is also sometimes a breakdown in communication between the rehabilitation team and the family doctor. General practitioners cannot be expected to make an informed decision about return to work if they have not been kept informed of the progress of their patient, but they are the health professionals that the patient knows best, and they are most likely to be approached about getting back to work.

What work should the patient go back to?

To the person who has had the head-injury, there is only one answer to this question, and that is to go back to the work that he was doing before the accident. Usually, however, there needs to be some compromise when he first goes back. This is because normally he will be starting work before he has made a complete recovery. In Chapter 5 we described some of the continuing effects of the injury. These effects put some constraints on how much he can do.

Firstly, because he is likely to tire quickly, the person will be unable to last out a full day when he starts back to work, and so the job has to be part-time. Related to this is how well he has regained control of the emotional system, because he will be more likely to lose control of his temper if he is over-tired. The rehabilitation team may suggest that the person should be given jobs where he does not have to deal with the public if this is likely to put him under pressure.

Next, because he will not be able to concentrate as well as he used to, the job needs to be structured to take into account his ability to concentrate. He will cope better if he does not have to work in noisy surroundings, for example, or where there is a lot to distract him. Because reaction times are likely to be slower than normal, he may not be safe using machinery, or driving a vehicle. If memory is not yet working well he needs to be given jobs where there will not be too many demands on memory, or where he can compensate by using memory aids. He will often have problems with balance, and so may need to avoid those parts of the job where he would need to work from ladders or scaffolding. Finally, as well as the head injury there are often other injuries which limit what work can be done.

In most cases one member of the team (usually the occupational therapist) will need to visit the workplace to check that the head-injured person will be able to manage.

How do we know whether or not the work trial is succeeding?

For most people the first few days at a new job or at a new school are very exciting. The excitement is great also for people who have had to take time off work because of a head injury. When they are eventually cleared to return to work the excess adrenalin will probably carry them through the first week. For this reason, we need to look at how they are doing three or four weeks after they go back, not how they did on the first three or four days.

The four parties who have a primary interest in the 'return-to-work' situation are the head-injured person, the employer, the rehabilitation team and the care-giver. All these people should be involved in the evaluation of the work trial. The team will usually set up a system for getting a weekly report from the employer, and they will modify the work hours depending on that report. Sometimes this does not happen, and the unfortunate head-injured person is stuck in a work trial which is too limited or too demanding for much longer than necessary because of this lack of supervision.

Sometimes the employer does not want to change the system, because as long as he or she has the head-injured person on a work trial wages do not have to be paid. The employer has no incentive to approach the rehabilitation team, the insurers, or the head-injured person to point out to them that the work trial does have an economic potential. In such a case an independent assessment of the work may be needed.

Although the person who has had the accident is the central character in the return-to-work arrangements, because of the head injury he is usually the least able to judge how he is doing. The basis of the problem of lack of insight was discussed in Chapter 5. Because of this the contribution from families or care-givers is very important. They will know if the person is over-tired when he gets home, or if he is becoming more irritable, restless, or aggressive at home. These are very clear signs that the hours of work should be cut back, and the rehabilitation team must be informed. The head-injured person may see this as a retrograde step, but the desire to spare his feelings should not stop the care-givers from doing this. The team members will explain that reducing the hours of a work trial does not mean that it was a failure. On the contrary, it is a sign of a successful trial where there is good communication between the people who are monitoring progress.

A system for returning to pre-injury employment or study

Planning for return to work or school will start before the injured person has reached the stage where the trial can begin. By the time that he is well enough to go back someone from the rehabilitation team will have visited the employer or teacher and will have explained the sorts of problems that the head injury has caused. Together they will have worked out what parts of the job he will be able to manage, and what changes will need to be made for him. If he normally works on a noisy factory floor, for example, he may need to start back in another area, say in the stockroom. Because it will be hard for the head-injured child to cope with the noise and bustle of a normal classroom, the school needs to arrange some quiet periods where he can have time out. Ideally, arrangements should be made for him to work with a tutor to catch up on work that has been missed.

It will have been explained to the employer or the teacher that the head-injured person will not be able to cope with a full day at work or school. It will also have been explained that he is likely to have some days where he may not be able to cope as well, or for as long, as he does on other days. Arrangements will have been made for him to have a place to lie down if he is unwell with a headache, or to leave early if necessary.

Starting small

When the person has made enough recovery to start back at work or school, a meeting will be set up with all the people involved; the head-injured person, the care-givers, the employer or teacher, and the rehabilitation team. The reason for this meeting is so that everyone is clear about the plans, and to arrange for systems to check how the trial is doing. Although it may seem to the person and the family that the trial is too restricted, the team members will explain that it is important to 'start small'. The team will stress that it is better to err on the side of caution when the hours of the trial are set. Two or three hours a day for two or three days a week are usually enough to start with, and these will be morning hours when he is most alert. The time will be built up only when it is clear that he can cope at home as well as at work.

Checking

Usually the rehabilitation team will continue to see the head-injured person on the days that he is not at work or school to monitor how he is doing. There will also be regular reviews of the hours, and regular contact with the employer or school teacher to make sure that any unexpected problems are dealt with. We have already explained the important part that the care-giver plays during this stage, in providing information on how well the person can cope when he is at home. A good return-to-work system will include families and care-givers in the review meetings. Sometimes the only change that needs to be made in work conditions is in the hours of work, because fatigue is such a limiting factor. Where part-time work or part-time attendance at school is something which has to be accepted as a long-term condition, it is important to remember that supervisors and school teachers will eventually change. The new people cannot be expected to know why the hours are restricted, or to understand the problems which the head-injured person has. It is important to make sure that if there is to be a change in personnel someone will be responsible for passing on information to the new person.

Alternative employment

We have already pointed out how people who tire more quickly and more deeply after head injury are limited in the number of hours that they can spend doing effective work. This problem also applies to the many cases where the head-injured person has not been able to go back to their old job, even on a part-time basis. However, before they get to this stage, they have already faced the problem of what work should they do instead? There are several obvious constraints. For example, if he has an arm or a leg that does not work very well the head-injured person cannot do a physically demanding job. If there are problems with thinking quickly or with remembering he will not be able to cope with a high-pressure job.

Once the person has accepted that he needs to change what he does for a living, he may be tempted to select a new occupation which is attractive but unrealistic. If he is advised that he will have to find a desk job, for example, he may opt for being an accountant when his aptitude is more suited to that of a clerk. We have already explained in Chapter 5 how head injury affects the ability to make complex decisions, and the person is usually not able on his own to judge which new occupation suits him best. Obviously his likes and dislikes need to be taken into account, but he also needs help from the family and from the rehabilitation team who will be able to judge whether or not he has the ability to retrain for a particular job.

Sometimes it is not only the unrealistic judgment of the head-injured person which guides the choice of an inappropriate new career.

If he and the family have always been high-achievers, it is difficult for them all to accept that the person must move to a less demanding job, or one which they see as of lower status. Unfortunately it is a fact that many people are left with permanent problems after a head injury that limit what job they can do. Families and care-givers need to realize that it is much kinder to their relative or friend to guide him to a job which he will be able to cope with, rather than to allow him to take on something in which he has no possibility of succeeding.

Some groups with special problems

Executives and managers

People in demanding and high-powered occupations have special difficulty getting back to work because the effect of head injury is to impair the skills which they need most. Decision making and ability to concentrate need to have recovered to a better level than for someone who has to return to a routine or repetitive job. So executives will have a longer period after injury before they can get back to work at all. Even the most secure person will be concerned about his position, and about what changes may have been made in his absence.

Executives and managers need special guidance to help them return to the work force, but they are understandably reluctant to have their employers and associates learn about the accident or the problems which it has caused. For this reason they need an experienced and authoritative counsellor who can help them rearrange their work schedule so that they will be able to cope. The most demanding meetings or appointments must be made for early in the day, for example, and they need to use their authority to defer important decisions until they have had enough time to consider them. They also need to accept and use any devices such as tape recorders which will take some of the load off their memory. Some executives have found that a special 'personal assistant' can be a help in keeping track of whether their energies are starting to flag, and can arrange the demands accordingly.

Finally, many people in this category are no longer young. In Chapter 7 we described how older people may not ever make a complete recovery. The possibility that the head-injured person may need to change to a less demanding job or to take early retirement needs to be faced.

The self-employed

Even when a person who is self-employed has adequate accident insurance it is often difficult for him to stay away from work for as long as he should. If the business is small there may not be anyone else with the skill which is needed to keep it going. If it is a larger concern he may worry about supervising the staff. If he has little or no insurance, financial difficulties may force him to try to cope at work before he is well enough to do this. In addition, he has the same problems as outlined in the last section for the executive.

Sometimes it may be possible for him to employ someone to take his place. Sometimes a better alternative may be to consider selling the business before it runs down because of his absence. Where possible, a business associate or friend should be brought in to help the head-injured person and the family reach the most sensible decision.

The unemployed

Although it may seem strange to talk about return to work for someone who does not have any work to return to, the unemployed person has special problems after he has had a head injury. This is because starting a work trial is an important stage of the rehabilitation process, and it is always more successful if it can be done in familiar surroundings at the place where the person was employed before the accident. If he has few or no work skills it may be difficult to find a place for him. If, as is often the case, he receives no accident insurance he may not be able to manage financially unless he finds paid work.

There are several problems in finding paid employment. Because of the head injury the person will be less likely to cope well with a job interview. He may not be able to answer questions quickly, or may not have regained social skills and the ability to judge how he is presenting himself. In addition, most employers prefer to take on someone who has not been off work for any length of time. When part of the period of unemployment is because of a head injury, the head-injured person is often even less acceptable as an employee.

The above-average student

Ability to learn and to concentrate is impaired after even minor head injuries. No matter how bright the student is this will affect his ability to cope with school. Although he has the advantage of an above-average store of knowledge, in most cases he has the disadvantage of never having had to work hard at his studies. He has not had to go over and over something that he wishes to learn in order to remember it later and it can be shattering for him to find that this is what he now needs to do. Compared to others in the class, he may now not learn things as quickly as expected. Compared to how he was before, the memory problem is very obvious.

Similar situations arise with other effects of the injury. Because he starts out with above-average ability, he may be able to cope with things at a good average level yet still be genuinely impaired by the accident. Where the problem is a severe one, so that he cannot even cope at an average level, a good student will need extra counselling. This is not just to help him to cope with the loss, but to help him re-direct his curricula so that he can make the best use of intact abilities.

The below-average student

Poor students also have special problems after a head injury. Because he has had poor academic records, it can be easy for families and teachers to miss that he has a genuine memory or language problem as a result of the head injury. If he was already 'learning-disabled', he will need to have a very severe memory problem before this is obvious in school performance. If he was a poor reader then the effect of damage to the parts of the brain that affect skills like reading will be less obvious.

Because the child has not done well at school, he will have less estab-lished learning to build on and to help compensate for these problems. He may also have lost the ability to take part in the non-academic school activities, such as sports, where the learning disability was not a handicap. Again, counselling is important to help the child understand why things are even harder for him and to guide him with alternative activities which he may be able to cope with.

Case histories

Samuel

Eventually the time came for Samuel to start attending classes at school again. This time things were very different. His tutor had worked with him on reading and maths, but he was still not able to do the work as well as before his accident, which meant he was well behind the other children in his class. Arrangements were made for him to work in the library with his tutor for these lessons. It was also accepted that he would go home at lunchtime for the first month, and again his grandmother came to stay to look after him. The orthopaedic specialist had cleared him to run, and he was able to take part in non-contact sports again.

Samuel enjoyed being back with his friends, and managed to get through the work he was given. His parents, his teacher, and his tutor knew that he was never going to be an academic person, and they focused on teaching the basic word and number skills that he would need as an adult. After the month was up he began to spend a full week at school. He coped with this apart from the occasional afternoon headache which he 'slept off' in the sick-bay. The tutor continued to work with him on his own, and the plan was that this would continue for the rest of the year.

Unfortunately things did not go as planned. The accident insurers were unwilling to continue to fund the tutor now that Samuel was back at school full-time, and asked for an independent specialist to review his case. The decision was that because he had already been behind in his school-work before the accident, the need for special schooling was not solely the result of his injury. The parents appealed against this decision, and provided a full report from Miss Jones pointing out that Samuel was much further behind his age group than he had been, but this made no difference. Rather than lose the tutor they decided to pay for his help themselves.

There were other set-backs. The first was when Samuel returned to hospital to have the pin taken out of his leg. The anaesthetic affected him badly, and for a while he had to return to spending just the morning at school. It took a couple of months for him to get back to where he had been before the surgery. The next crisis was when he moved from the junior school he had been attending to high school. All students had to take an entrance exam, and Samuel was placed in a class for 'slow learners'. This would have been appropriate except that the other children in the class had severe learning disabilities, and Samuel hated it. However, by now his parents knew what was needed, and were able to arrange for him to be in a higher level class and join the 'slow learners' only for maths and language lessons.

By the time Samuel had finished his schooling he had had several attempts, supervised by his neurologist, to stop taking the anti-convulsants, and had accepted that if he wanted to be able to drive a car and to earn a living he needed to make sure that he did not have any more seizures. By now, taking his medication had become part of his daily routine and, apart from the scar on his thigh, was the only evidence that he had ever been in an accident.

Jonas

Because Jonas had such a short time left to complete his carpentry apprenticeship it was hoped that he could work these hours and obtain his qualification, even if it was unlikely that he would ever be able to work as a carpenter again. After the tension that trying to work on his car had caused, it was decided to put this plan on hold and find some alternative work that he could do. This was hard as all his skills had been in technical and mechanical subjects, and all his interest had been in the building field.

The first placement was in a local builder's supply store. The manager agreed that he could spend a few hours on alternate mornings as a work trial, provided that Stephen came with him to monitor what he was doing. Jonas enjoyed the environment and was sure that this was a first step to getting back to the work force. With Stephen's help he was able to find his way round the store, and also to find the cashier where he was to take customers and the goods that they needed. He rarely needed the cashier however, as he could not accept that people came to the shop not to talk with him, but because they needed some items, often in a hurry. He was then tried in the stock room, but again was too easily distracted and also too disruptive, and after three weeks the work trial was ended.

At this time some of the buildings at the rehabilitation centre were being painted. The two painters working on the job were older men, and were kind hearted as well as tolerant. They felt sorry for Jonas, and agreed that he could spend some time with them. He helped with sanding and preparing the walls, and under their supervision worked on areas he could reach from ground level. Soon he had slipped into a routine of working with the painters every morning, and by the time they had finished the contract he had decided that being a painter was what he wanted to do.

The accident insurer's representative on Jonas's case was aware that he had no economic potential at this stage, and there was no problem continuing to pay his full weekly compensation. Once this was sorted out the painters arranged to take him to work with them whenever they had jobs which would be suitable. The only problems were that

Jonas did tend to make personal and sometimes offensive comments about the occupants of the houses they were working on, but both painters quickly learned how to distract him with another task, and also to make sure that before they started any new contract they had warned the owners that Jonas was not always polite or tactful.

The next step, now that he had an occupation that he enjoyed and was settled in, was to move from the unit at the rehabilitation centre. The team agreed that Jonas could not be expected to cope on his own, and that he had managed at the supervised living unit only because Stephen had been there with him. However, this support could not be provided any longer, and the unit was needed for another patient. Thus the decision was made to try a small supervised accommodation complex which had been established for accident survivors who could not manage on their own. At first Jonas was not very enthusiastic, but was won over when he found that the complex included both a swimming pool and a games room. There were five units in the complex, all completely self-contained, and a full time warden and his wife to make sure that each tenant was coping. This worked well, especially as one of 'his' painters lived within walking distance so he was able to easily get to work with him.

Jonas never finished his apprenticeship. He continued to help the painters until one of them collapsed with a heart attack, and the other decided to retire. This was a bad time for Jonas, but eventually the warden's wife found him a placement with another painter. He never returned to driving a car, and never managed to get paid employment. Apart from a period of just over a year when he had moved in with a woman he had met and fallen for, he lived permanently at the complex. His friend visited him once a month so that he could see the daughter born as a result of their brief liaison. He was happy with his life.

Pauline

The partners in her law firm were all pleased with the work that Pauline had been producing, and were eager to have her return to work. They were prepared to have her work part-time, not just because they felt responsible for her accident since it had happened while she was at work, but also because she was a valuable member of the staff. Working only half days did limit what she could do, and she was not able to take on any of the court work that she had always enjoyed. However, she was so pleased to be back that she willingly took on every case she was given. The first two or three weeks left her exhausted, so that she had almost no energy to drive herself home at midday, but eventually she learned to pace herself, and to plan her morning schedules more carefully.

As she had done when she was working at home, she continued to test herself every now and then, but after six months could still not cope with more than five hours at the office. The senior partner was happy to have her do whatever hours she could, but Pauline was aware that some of the other staff were getting annoyed that they had to take on half her work. She overheard comments about it being almost a year since the accident, and that she had not even needed to be admitted to hospital so she could not have been that bad.

She worried about this so much that she began to have disturbed nights and as a result began to find it hard to handle even five hours. Finally John insisted on another visit with the counsellor and the senior partner. He agreed to the suggestion that they restructure her position and employ someone to job-share with her, and emphasized that this would continue for as long or as short a time as was needed. Pauline eventually built up her time to six hours a day, but never managed to work effectively for longer than that.

Nor did her relationship ever return to the comfortable and exciting partnership it had been before the accident. She realized that she did not have the energy to do anything about this, and eventually accepted that this was as good as things were going to be. John took longer to come to terms with this. Their lives drifted slowly but not dramatically apart.

10 Long-term adjustment

It is a sad fact that not all head-injured patients will recover well enough for return to work or school ever to be considered. Even if these people carefully follow all the advice given in the last chapter, and even if they have extremely supportive families and employers, if they do not get back the mental and physical skills which they need to function in full open employment they will never be able to take this step.

If you have read this book through from the beginning, you will know by now that recovery from head injury can often take many years. It is also important to realize that recovery may never be complete. At some stage you and your family member or friend may need to come to terms with this and to accept that the life which you all had before the accident is over. This is a step which you must take before you can all alter your expectations and set up some more realistic goals for yourselves.

It is very difficult to come to terms with this incomplete recovery. You may feel that you are giving up hope, and also that, in a sense, you are letting down the person who had the accident. But until you and the injured person do make adjustments, you run the risk of building up unnecessary frustration, because if your expectations of what the future will bring are unrealistic you are really setting up your friend or family member for failure. This chapter outlines some of the steps that may help you to work through this difficult period. Note, however, that this advice cannot replace individual counselling from someone who knows your special circumstances. It is important that you talk to your family doctor about how you can get this special help.

Letting go

One of the most difficult things about accepting that the accident has put an end to the life which your family member or friend might have had is that he *is* still alive. If the worst had happened, and he had died, you would by now have gone through the grieving process. You would have had the opportunity to mourn his passing, with a funeral where you, your family, and friends could pay tribute to him, and you could publicly acknowledge that he had gone from you. But you cannot do that now. You can see the 'old' person every day. Even if the patient is unable to walk or communicate, he has the same shaped face, the same hair colour, and he may have some of the same mannerisms, maybe the same glint in the eye when he is being stubborn. This is certainly not a stranger who has taken the place of the person you knew and loved. This 'new' character, however, has lost many of the things which made up the old life. You all need to accept these losses, and to get on with making a new life.

When should you make this decision? We have already said that it may seem that you are giving up. You may also feel that if you do not keep pushing, and your friend or family member stops trying, then he will not have any chance to recover. But we are not advising that you and he sit back and say, 'Well, this is it. This is how it is always going to be.' What 'letting go' means is that you need to let go of the things from the life before the accident that are impossible for the person now. The ideal time for this to take place is as soon as you are able to come to terms with the fact that there have been these losses. Later on we shall discuss how you can help the person to let go too, but for now we will concentrate on you, the person who is the care-giver.

Your relative or friend may have been keen on sports but may have had no interests outside the sport of his choice. However, no amount of will power will allow him to run a marathon with paralysed legs, or if he is still uncoordinated and has poor balance. Having 'running in the marathon' as the goal is unrealistic in either case. It will also hinder him from looking around for other activities or interests which could be practical and possible for him to do now. You and he need to let go of the person who was a budding marathon champion, and work at a level which is appropriate now for someone with his handicaps. This advice applies equally to the law student who cannot speak clearly, to the apprentice who has lost the ability to control his hands, or to the artist who has lost his sight. You need to let go of the person who had the potential to follow these careers.

We have already talked about the way head injury affects mood and temperament. We have explained how fatigue can be a persistent problem, and how the sleep cycle can be disturbed. We have also explained how making decisions can be more difficult, and how the person may no longer be able to appreciate the effect on others of what he does and says. All these things make up 'personality', and it is not surprising that families often talk about how the injury has changed their relative's personality. In the sense that personality can be defined by the sum of the ways that we react to the things which happen to us, then if he reacts differently to the way he would have done before the accident, your relative or friend does have a different personality now. But this does not mean that he is a different person. Although it may be hard to do, you will find that you cope much better with the effects of the accident once you can let go of the pre-injury personality, and accept that your partner or relative or friend now reacts in a different way.

All this is easier for you to accept than it is for the person who has had the head injury. We all have a picture of ourselves and the sort of person that we are. Psychologists call this our self-image. We suspect that it takes a long time for the self-image to change after a head injury. Even if he needs to use wheelchairs to get around, for example, and has problems making other people understand what he says, or reacts irrationally at times, a head-injured person will resent being placed in a facility for physically handicapped or psychiatric patients because he does not see himself as disabled. Neither does he have anything in common with the other patients. For a long time people who have had a head injury still consider themselves to be young, healthy, and able; a person who happens to have had an accident, so at the moment needs to use a wheelchair.

> We need to realize that for a long time head-injured people still think of themselves as they were before their accidents

It is important for you and his friends and relatives to remember that this is how the person sees himself. To him, he is as physically attractive, as witty and the same good company as he was before his injury. Unhappily, it is obvious to those around him that he is not, and people naturally respond very differently to the 'new' person that he has become. Indeed, very often embarrassing or unacceptable behaviour can be interpreted by those around him as a desperate attempt on his part to prove that he is the same old self, because of the way others now respond to him. We said earlier that we would talk about ways to help your relative or friend come to terms with the fact that the accident has changed him, and that he needs to change what he expects to get out of life. In essence this means that we need to get him to face up to the fact that the self-image which he carries from the days before the accident is no longer accurate. This does not mean that you get him to replace it with the negatives of 'failure, crippled, ugly, or useless'. It is for this very reason that you, the rehabilitation staff, and the counsellors will have tried to find something that he can succeed at to replace the things that he can no longer do. This is simply what is meant by the advice to set realistic goals. You need to help him feel good about himself because of the things that he can do, not bad because of the things that he cannot do. We cannot stress too strongly that you need to make sure that he has appropriately trained counsellors to help him through this.

You, as the non head-injured person in your relationship, will need to work out the changes that your family member or friend will have to make, as well as the changes which you must make yourself. You may also have to act as a back-up counsellor for him. Again, this is a difficult role, especially if he is a parent or partner. It is worth repeating the advice that we gave earlier, that is, do not be too proud to ask relatives and friends for their help and support.

Eventually you will reach the stage where you are ready to accept the fact that the accident has changed what you can expect from your loved one. There are many different emotions that you will feel on the way to this acceptance. Before we talk about ways in which you can handle some of these emotions, it is important to remember that these are perfectly natural reactions to the losses which you have had. It is at this stage that you and your family most need support from your local head-injury group, and reassurance that there are other people who have been through the same process.

Grief

We have already pointed out that when a person does not survive a head injury, family and friends are able to grieve for him, and eventually to move on to life without him. It is important to remember that you need to grieve also for the things which the accident has taken away from you, even though you have not physically lost him. It is normal and natural to be sad that your relative or friend is so different from the way he was before the injury. It is normal and natural to be sad that he can no longer be the companion who was able to share the interests which you had. It is normal and natural to be sad that you have lost the support of your partner or parent. You need to accept also that it is all right to cry. Probably at this stage the person will not be ready to let go of the way he was before the accident. Neither will he be ready to grieve. But you can. You are allowed to cry for what you have lost. Do not feel guilty that this somehow implies that you are crying because he survived, and that you wish that he had died rather than be left with such handicaps. Do not feel guilty that you are being self-indulgent and should be able to 'keep a stiff upper lip'. Crying can be a very good safety valve.

Work through your grief
Allow yourself to cry
Allow yourself to remember the past
Allow others to talk about the past
Accept that the past is behind you
Accept that the future will be different

When you get to this stage you need to allow yourself some time alone when you can weep for what has gone, and when you have the opportunity re-live, through photographs and mementoes, how things were before the accident. Some people find that it also helps to make a list of the things which have been lost, or to put together in one album a record of your friend or relative's sporting or academic achievements. The important thing to realize is that the list and the album are from the past, that they are from the different life that you had before the accident. You also need to encourage his friends to talk to you about the things which your relative or friend used to say and do. Finally, encourage other members of the family to talk about the things which you all did together, and that the head-injured person will not be able to do again. It is not morbid to appreciate the past and to mourn for it. It may be that having a good cry together will help you all.

Anger

Anger is a common and natural response following a head injury. We are all familiar with this 'why me?' type of anger. Many of the losses which a head injury brings about are very hard to accept and anger can be an issue for your friend or relative throughout his rehabilitation. Most often the anger is expressed against close relatives and friends, not because they deserve it, but because they are most trusted. By this we mean that it is safe for him to be himself when he is with people he relies on for support. When he is away from home he may be able to make the extra effort and hide his anger from acquaintances or employers. If he showed this anger too often with them it might lead to rejection or loss of employment. For relatives and care-givers this can be hurtful, and they need to understand that this does not mean lack of respect or love on his part.

In our experience the 'anger phase' is just that — a phase which will generally pass. In the meantime if anger is a problem in your family here are a few suggestions that may help. If the anger is so strongly expressed that it spills over, or risks spilling over into actual hurt to others, then seek professional help. Try not to read motives into every angry outburst. There is often no real intent behind the anger, no plan or scheme. He may not seem like the person you knew before the accident but it is too early to think in terms of 'changed personality'. Personality changes, though they can occur, are much less frequent than you might suppose. Try to think of the anger as temporary and separate from the person you know and love.

Ask yourself if you are being too helpful, for this can sometimes be a trigger for his frustration. It is easy to get stuck in the groove of helping and guiding and taking responsibility away from him. Though this may be necessary in the early stages of recovery it can be irritating for him later on as he tries to regain control over his life and wishes to make his own choices. Avoid arguments, but discuss important differences when both you and he are fresh and calm. Remember that it often makes no sense to him either that he finds trivial things so irritating. Finally, as we pointed out earlier, anger is often simply the result of fatigue.

Dealing with anger
The anger phase won't last
Don't pursue arguments
Think of the anger as separate. Don't take the hurt to heart
Find a safe outlet for anger (e.g. physical activity and exercise)

Your friend or relative will also experiment with different ways of coping with anger and frustration. Physical activity and exercise is helpful to many people as is 'getting away from it all' for a quiet period. Others have found some benefit from relaxation techniques. There are no easy solutions and things which work for other people may not work for the person with a head injury. The problem is usually one of unpredictable flashes of anger rather than an attitude problem.

Guilt

What parent or partner of a head-injured person has not spent time agonizing over casual remarks and complaints made ages in the past, which taken out of context suggest that the person was a nuisance and that a head injury is the least that they deserve? This reaction may occur partly because of the very human need to find an explanation for the dreadful thing that has happened. There has to be a reason why he was the one struck by a bus, and why you are being punished. It is the rare relationship where there was never any resentment on one side or the other, however momentarily, at some time in the past.

It is hard to forgive yourself for these remarks, but you need to leave your guilt outside the door and bring your normal rational mind into play. How many times have you snapped at your friend or relative, or carped, or unfairly accused him of something? Was he punished with a head injury each time? Of course he was not. Why, when most of your thoughts about your partner or family member have been positive, would one instance when you lost your temper have resulted in him being 'struck down' like this. Further, what sort of mechanism would need to be involved if every negative complaint about a person resulted in a head injury?

Sometimes assuming guilt allows us to cope with awful things like the effects of a head injury, and to find a 'reason' why it has happened. The problem is that this interferes with your relationship with your loved one. If you accept that you are to blame for their condition, then you are going to treat him in a different way to normal, and so you have doubly lost him. He is also likely to react differently to you if you treat him as someone that you have damaged. Again this may reinforce your sense of guilt.

Many people feel responsible for the injury because indirectly the person was in a position to be hurt because of something that they did or did not do. Maybe the motor cycle that a son crashed on was a birthday present from his parents. Maybe the son was able to buy the hang-glider that he rode into a cliff only because his parents lent him the money. Maybe a husband was driving his car that night because his wife had asked him to collect their daughter from the school social.

Guilt is very much an emotional response. Common sense tells us that we are only responsible for the head injuries of those we have run down in cars, struck down with blunt weapons, or where we have in other ways directly inflicted the damage. Some few of us may be responsible for a person's injuries. For the others it is important to accept the principle of cause and effect, and to accept that no amount of taking the blame on yourself is going to alter what has happened already. The only sure consequence of acting the guilty party is that you will be a less effective care-giver.

Blame

We have talked about the problems of taking on the responsibility yourself for the injuries that your family member has suffered. It is even more important to refrain from unfairly putting the blame on somebody else. The only advantage of having someone to blame is that it somehow 'makes sense' of what has happened. However, the price that you pay for this is out of all proportion. In some cases the person who is unfairly blamed is a family member or friend. Every one of the head-injured person's associates is affected by the injury, and he or she needs the support of every one during the recovery stage. If one parent blames the other for letting their son borrow the family car, and therefore for the accident, their relationship will be strained and their ability to support their son compromised. If the parents blame their son's wife for encouraging his interest in polo, and therefore for the accident, it will be their son who is damaged by the family rift. If the family blame the friend who let their son have a spin on his new motor cycle, and hold him responsible for the accident, they will not only reinforce his own guilt, but it will make it impossible for the friend to offer the support which he would like to give.

But there are many cases where responsibility for the accident is very clear. What about the careless driver who rounded a corner on the wrong side of the road? What about the drunk who drove through a red light? What about the fairground operator who sold rides on dangerous equipment? What about the construction company which did not make sure that building materials would not fall on passers by? Obviously they are all responsible for the accidents which followed, and there are two stages which your need to find someone to blame will pass through. The first stage is retribution. The guilty party must be caught and punished. Taken to the extreme, this can be quite destructive. You can be so obsessed by the knowledge that the guilty party has not yet been found or arrested that you neglect the needs of the head-injured person and of the other members of your family. Even after the police have at last found him or her, although this gives you tremendous satisfaction, you cannot relax. Waiting for the court case and the sentence gives you the opportunity to let your imagination run riot. You know what you would do if it was up to you; you are obsessed by the need to punish, and your every interaction with the victim feeds this obsession.

> There is no punishment that can be given to someone who has caused a head injury that will alter the effects of that injury

The second stage is healthier. Here you want to make sure that the culprits or people like them will not be able to hurt others in the same way that they have hurt your head-injured relative or friend. Depending on your personality you may become an activist or a joiner, but you will want laws against drinking and driving, better safety standards, and so on. This stage fills a very real need, and it is important that you find an avenue for this kind of protest. Indeed, people who can identify a guilty party and a contributing set of circumstances which can be changed can cope better with being involved with someone who has had a severe head injury. It takes away the senselessness of the accident if you can see that because it happened some good will come. To some extent this gives you back the feeling of control over the destinies of you and your loved one, which the accident had shattered.

Unfortunately, having someone to blame sometimes means that people are trapped in the past, and do not move on to learning how to cope with the present or the future. Having someone to blame, having a focus for our anger, may satisfy our need to understand why the accident happened. It stops us taking on unnecessary guilt or unfairly ascribing blame to other relatives or friends. But it does not necessarily mean that we are then able to come to terms with the accident. It is easy to slip into a blind alley, the 'if only' mode. If only I had not given him that motor cycle. If only you had not asked him to run that errand. If only that drunk or careless driver had not been on the road.

If only that roller coaster had been condemned. This kind of response to the effects of head injury in your relative or family member is as pointless as the search for guilt or blame. Eventually we have to accept that we are not able to turn the clock back. We have to accept that apportioning guilt, or accepting blame, will not change the outcome of the head injury one iota. In the same way, whether the drunken driver whose car went through a red light and hit your daughter is sent to jail for 20 years, or fined a trivial amount, will not alter the course of her recovery. On the other hand, if you are able to accept that how you respond to the culprit's sentence can play a vital part in determining how well your daughter responds, you have made great strides towards understanding how you can help her cope with the effects of head injury. We have stressed the importance of looking forward, of making plans for the future and not mourning forever for the past. As long as you are in the 'if only' mode you will not be able to move on to this stage of looking forward.

Denial

One way of coping with an unpleasant fact is to deny that it exists. This is hard to do if the effects of the accident are easily seen, such as a paralysis or a persistent coma, or if the effects are very obvious, such as difficulty with speech. In these cases it is often the poor likelihood of recovery which is denied. If you deny that he will never be completely better, you do not have to worry about how your friend or relative will manage. Indeed, in the early stages, this coping mechanism is very important in helping you to maintain your sanity.

Eventually, however, the time will come when you have to accept the reality of the situation. It is where denial persists beyond this point that it can interfere with your ability to come to terms with what has happened, and to make the adjustments to your own life that have to be made. You need to work through your anger and guilt and the other emotions which we have talked about, but you cannot do this as long as you deny that there is cause for these emotions, because you pretend that everything will be all right.

Denial is also often used as a coping mechanism further on down the track, when there may have been reasonably good physical recovery but the person continues to have memory, concentration, and behavioural problems. This is when it is tempting to refuse to accept that the recovery is not complete. A young man's parents may seize on an instance when he forgot something in the past, for example, as evidence that 'His memory has always been awful', or use excuses such as 'Well he has never been able to concentrate' or 'He has never been interested in things like that' to explain why he has difficulty with simple tasks. It easier for them to handle the evidence that his behaviour is inappropriate or embarrassing by seeing this as an extension of how he acted in the past. 'He always had a droll sense of humour', or 'He was never a conventional person'.

The problem is that this denial often coincides with the period, described in Chapter 5, in which the patients themselves lack insight or awareness of the problems which they have. We have explained how family and friends can help them through this stage by showing them where they make mistakes, and how they can correct them. If families as well as patients deny that there are any problems, no rehabilitation facility will be able to help them overcome the problems. Families who have been through this often comment that they had reached a point when they were sick of hospitals, therapists, and the accident. They wanted to carry on with life, to put the accident behind them and pretend that it had not happened. Later on, when it becomes too obvious to deny that everything is not back to normal, or when the head-injured person himself becomes more realistic, the family are ready to get back into the recovery system. The need for 'time out' can sometimes be averted if counselling and support is kept up well beyond the early weeks after the injury.

We have looked at some of the emotions that families and caregivers need to work through as they progress towards setting up satisfactory programmes for their head-injured relative. There are three areas of change. The final sections in this chapter look at the changes that need to be made to the person's family life, to his social life, and to his work life.

The new family life

Where the head-injured person is an adult son or daughter, the change from independence to dependence brings an equally drastic change to the parents' lifestyle. After some 20 years rearing a family, the parents have reached a time when they are probably more financially secure than they have ever been, and when they have their home to themselves for the first time since their early married days. Then the accident happens, and they eventually bring their injured son or daughter home. Once again the parents have a dependent person to care for, and they have to face the fact that the days when they had only themselves to please have gone. Parents also have to face the fact that they need to plan for a future when they may be too old or infirm to provide the care which the son or daughter may need.

Although the parents are returned to the role of care-givers, and the adult to the role of dependent child, the situation is not the same as it had been the first time round. The head-injured person has usually spent several years as an adult earning his own living and looking after himself, and so the new family life demands adjustments on both sides. However, because the parents are the ones with the means and mobility to do things, it is often they who decide what the adjustment should be.

The head-injury families who function best are those who, through trial and error, evolve a system where the needs for care and dependency are balanced by two other important needs — the need for privacy, and the need for some control over the situation. Both the cared-for and the care-givers need to have some time on their own. Where circumstances allow, this can be managed by modifying the family home so that the head-injured person has his or her own private apartment. However, even if this is not practical, privacy need not only be possible within the four walls of the bedroom. Family or volunteers can be organized to take the person for the whole day once a week, for example, so that the parents can have time to themselves, or to entertain or visit their own friends. Similarly, the parents can arrange to be out of the house for set times so that their son or daughter can entertain friends without them.

The other need for both parties is the need to have some control over what is happening. There may be a great deal that the head-injured person has no control over because of the accident. If he cannot move around without assistance, for example, the times when he gets out of bed or shifts from one room to the next have to depend on when a care-giver is available to help him. However, even the most severely disabled person should be given the opportunity to make as many decisions as are practical about his life. Depending on circumstances, these decisions may range from when he has his meals and what he has to eat to the disposal of income. Eventually the parents must accept that their dependent child needs to be given the right to decide what happens to him, and that he also needs to get back the right to make mistakes if that is how the decisions turn out.

> **The dependant in a head-injury family needs**
> Care
> Privacy
> Control
>
> **The care-givers in a head-injury family need**
> Support
> Privacy
> Control

We have focused on the most typical case, that in which the head-injured person is young and single. The special problems that arise when he is a partner or parent have already been discussed in Chapter 7. How well your family is able to develop a new life after the accident depends not only on how willing you are as the care-giver to adapt to a changed role in this 'new' family. It also depends on whether or not the head-injured person is able to modify his role and adjust to the changes that the accident has brought about.

The new social life

Probably one of the saddest secondary effects of a severe head-injury is loneliness. In the first weeks after the injury there is usually no short-age of friends to visit the person. The tragedy of the accident is very fresh, and the 'old' person still very real. Gradually, as the months go by, the situation changes. The frequency of visits drops rapidly. This may be because of communication problems. Talking with the head-injured person may be such an effort that it becomes easier to put off this effort until another day. It may be because of the changed way in which he reacts. It can be very painful for friends to see their old com-panion behaving in an atypical way. It will also be because, as time goes by, the old friends will have met new people and they will have had new experiences that they cannot share with their friend. We all grow apart from acquaintances that we do not see regularly. When your life is in the outside world where you earn your living and pursue the leisure activities which interest you, it is not surprising that the only thing which you have in common with your old friend, whose life is confined to the hospital or rehabilitation center, is life before the acci-dent. It is not surprising, therefore, that there is less and less contact with old friends.

New friends are difficult to find. This applies not only to the severely disabled head-injury victim, but also to the person who has regained the ability to walk and to talk. The reasons are easy to understand. We have stressed the problems which he may have with tiredness, irritability, coping with noise, or with crowds. It is not surprising that he has difficulty coping with social gatherings too; thus it is not surprising that invitations to social gatherings eventually dry up.

Community groups which have been organized to provide social activities for the disabled are not always the answer to the problem. We have discussed the long lag that there is before the head-injured person sees himself as other than an able-bodied person. The denial mechanism we described earlier in the chapter is relevant there. Reactions to people with special needs will typically be of denial, and he may refuse to accept that he also has these needs. This is partly because the only common ground between the traumatically and congenitally disabled is the disability. Until the accident the trauma victim was able to participate in many activities that he can no longer cope with. Yet he will retain his interests in, for example, sport and fast cars. The interests of the congenitally disabled will, of necessity, be very different.

> The traumatically and the congenitally disabled have little in common except the disability.

Community groups which provide venues for social activities especially for head-injured people and their families seem to work better, possibly because they feel more comfortable among people who understand the problems which they have. However, there is the obvious disadvantage that this restricts their social life to the company of others like themselves.

Some people find friends outside this circle among two different age groups. They may often find it easy to relate to the elderly, who also cannot keep up the fast pace of doing things that the peers of the head-injured person expect. They may also often find company among younger children, who are usually delighted to find an adult who has the time to spend hours on end talking to them about a favourite subject.

The new work life

Although it is unlikely that the survivor of a very severe head injury will ever be able to return to full-time paid employment, he has the same need as everyone else to be productive. This need is recognized by most agencies, but it is not always met successfully. Sheltered workshops provide something to do to fill in the waking hours, but often the occupation that head-injured persons are given is not something which they find interesting, or that gives them satisfaction.

We believe that even when a person can cope with some of the activities in a sheltered workshop, if he does not enjoy this work then it is not the appropriate place for him. In other words, the need to feel satisfied at the end of the day with what has been achieved outweighs the convention that he should receive payment for what he does. This means that the new work life does not necessarily mean paid employment. Neither should the new work life entail a nine-to-five job, as it is likely that the person will not have the ability to concentrate for that period of time and would get too tired to do anything else if he did.

The task that he does should depend on his abilities and his interests. The next chapter looks at the type of rehabilitation service which would be provided in an ideal world. Vocational rehabilitation is an important part of that service, and we would hope that your relative or friend will have the help of a specialist in vocational rehabilitation to help him to discover what the new work in his new work life will be.

11 Providing a head-injury service

Up to now we have been talking about the effects of head injury and how the problems are dealt with. We have agreed that many of the problems are very difficult to solve. Though nowadays the standard of acute medical care is usually good, we have also suggested that the other services that the authorities provide are often inadequate, both because they have not understood what is needed and because they have not given the requirements of head-injured people enough priority in their budgets.

In this chapter we will try to summarize the problems of management and suggest what a good head-injury service should provide. We will then look at the difficulties from the point of view of the people who have to provide the service so that we can argue with them on their own terms. Lastly, we will suggest ways in which concerned people can influence the decision makers.

The problems of management

We will list the outstanding problems of management in the order in which most people meet them as the person who has had the accident goes through the stages from the emergency department onwards.

1. *Information and relations with staff*. Families and close friends need to know what is happening and to be able to ask questions about the issues that are important to them. This runs through the whole time span.

   Action: There must be a charter for management at all stages which insists on regular opportunities as of right for the family to be told what is happening and for them to have questions answered.

2. *Support and understanding*. Like the previous section but looking at the more personal side of relationships. In the first stages the family need counselling and support in their grief and anxiety. Later the

person who was injured and their family need to understand the problems which each of them has, as far as they can, and to make allowances for each other. This is needed for those who have had mild injuries and persisting problems as well as for those with major injuries.

Action: Three sources of help can be used. Firstly, counselling by professionals must be available in the early stages of grief and anxiety. However, families are often too upset and not ready for it at this stage, and it should be offered again as often as it seems needed. Secondly, again at a later stage, support is often welcomed from families who have gone through the same problems themselves. Lastly, those who have themselves been injured and have recovered can sometimes explain the situation with more authority than anyone. The first, professional, counselling needs to be organized by the acute hospital. Later counselling may be provided by the hospital, by voluntary agencies and by head-injury societies, but professional guidance and monitoring should always be available.

3. *Hospital services in the acute stage.* Most hospitals accept the need for a special trauma service and try to organize as good a one as their situation allows. Small country hospitals have special problems and for severe injuries most rely on regional services and use skilled transport teams to get patients to expert centres. When the life-threatening stage is over, after one or two months, the situation is often much less satisfactory. Many hospitals have to keep such patients in an acute treatment setting, which is not geared to their rehabilitation needs. Others transfer them to long-stay facilities, sometimes primarily geriatric, which are not geared to rehabilitation needs.

Action: Hospitals need to provide accommodation for patients whose primary need is acute rehabilitation but who still need some medical and nursing care and are not fit to leave hospital.

Management needs — first stage
A trauma service expert in managing head injury
Information and support, as of right, whenever needed

---

4. *Rehabilitation services on discharge from hospital.* In many places these are limited. Expertise may not be available. The amount of treatment that is offered each week may be below the level at which it

is effective. This may be because of a lack of staff or facilities or there may be difficulty in transport to the rehabilitation centre with shorter hours of treatment and extra fatigue.

Action: It must be possible for rehabilitation to occupy the major part of the week, without unnecessary fatigue. If it is needed, live-in accommodation must be available.

Management needs — second stage
Expert rehabilitation services:
in hospital
live-in rehabilitation
out-patient rehabilitation
rehabilitation is a full time job

---

5. *Return to normal occupation*. It must be the aim to return every injured person to their previous occupation, or failing this to the highest level of earning or personal satisfaction possible. Existing vocational rehabilitation organizations are often unaware of the special needs of the head-injured person or may be unable to supply the extra facilities needed.

Action: Vocational rehabilitation centres must provide staff and expertise, with the other facilities needed, to rehabilitate people with head injuries.

6. *Job opportunities*. Someone who has had a head injury often cannot be found work. This may be because they are less tolerant of fatigue or stress, or because there are behavioural problems. Much of the difficulty is due to prejudice and lack of cooperation on the part of employers.

Action: Employers must be persuaded that a person who has had a head injury has a worthwhile potential, provided that allowances are made for them. They should be given incentives to provide work in which the head-injured person can be employed to the profit of the employer and the advantage of the employee.

7. *Occupation for a person for whom a job cannot be found*. Some people who have had head injuries will not be able to work in a commercial environment because of physical, intellectual or behavioural problems. Someone in this position needs an occupation as a source of satisfaction, to give structure to their days and to provide them with social relationships.

Action: From a drop-in centre to sheltered workshops, a range of opportunities is needed for people who cannot work in a normal environment. Some of these opportunities are best supplied by voluntary agencies such as head-injury societies, others such as sheltered workshops need institutional or government support. No-one should be left to linger at home with nothing to do and no-one to meet because of the lack of these facilities.

Management needs — third stage
Vocational rehabilitation
Job opportunity
A place with dignity and satisfaction for those without a job

---

8. *Major behavioural problems*. A few people who have had head injuries are left with major problems of behaviour which need full-time professional care, either for treatment in the expectation of return to independent living or occasionally for long-term care. This is a psychiatric problem, but in many places psychiatric services are unable to supply the sort of care that is needed.
   Action: Psychiatric services are needed for people with serious behavioural problems following head injury, to make it possible for them to live in the community, or failing this in safety with reasonable dignity and comfort.

9. *Persisting problems with mild head injuries*. It is becoming recognized that 5–10 per cent of people who have had a mild head injury have difficulties in getting back to normal function and employment, and that their problems may last from a few weeks to several years. In many places there are not the psychological and medical services to deal with their problems.
   Action: Mild head-injury clinics should be available to the accident services of all but the smallest hospital centres.

Management needs — areas often neglected
Severe behavioural problems
Mild head injury
Do not let people with head injury be written off

Presenting needs to the authorities

In many places the needs of head-injured people are not being met. Some parts of the service as we have outlined it above may not be available, and often there is no central organization to make sure that everyone works together. Anyone who goes to a meeting of head-injured people and their families will realize that there is a majority of dissatisfied customers.

The authorities that run accident and rehabilitation services vary from place to place, but the arguments that affect them are likely to be the same everywhere. They will take some humane notice of the amount of suffering experienced, but they will need other reasons to give priority to any area. Usually they will be most influenced by the cost of any extensions of their existing service and they will not agree to any increase in funding unless it can be shown that obvious gains can be set against this. In preparing an argument, the first need therefore is to know the numbers and severities of the injuries in your community, with an estimate of the human cost: deaths, family disruptions, days off work, and any other information you can supply.

The authority will need a reason for priority. It may say that it cannot single out one service for improvement. You can then argue that head injury is a consequence of the modern way of living, and that therefore the community has a special responsibility. You can point out that there is no doubt that the community inherits special problems when head injuries are poorly rehabilitated, in the shape of long-term disability and the need to make provision for people whose thinking and behaviour remain disturbed.

Economic arguments will be powerful. It will be relevant to have an estimate of the current cost of handling head injuries, and to make a reasonable prediction of savings that might be made by improving the service. The inefficiency of using acute hospital beds for long-term care, and the saving from provision of less expensive rehabilitation beds is a good argument in some places. It is more difficult to give exact figures for reduction of the period of disability which can result from good rehabilitation, but the general argument can be put forcefully. This may be more telling when dealing with insurers, who bear the burden of long disability, rather than with the hospital authorities.

Some figures from Auckland, New Zealand, may be useful as an illustration and a starting point. These come from a survey in a city of 850 000 people, and are comparable with figures reported in the USA and UK.

Figures for numbers of head injuries and hospital use from a survey in Auckland, New Zealand, in 1986
These are expressed in number per 100 000 of population per year

Admitted to hospital
with a primary diagnosis of head injury	65
with a head injury and severe multiple injuries	5.4
with other injuries but also a head injury	57

Seen at hospital but not admitted	654
Hospital bed-days occupied — primary head injury and severe multiple injuries	4,700
With persisting problems after mild head injury (2/3 with problems lasting more than a month)	30

Lastly, the professionals who are involved should be mobilized to help. This together with strong public pressure can produce results. The Royal College of Physicians of London commissioned a report on physical disability in young people which has been very influential. In 1986 it made strong recommendations on the need for services for head-injured people, particularly for a central organizing body in each area. Many other professional bodies in the UK, the USA, Australia and elsewhere have made similar recommendations. The way that public support can be organized and who can be persuaded to lend themselves to a movement of this sort will be different in every area. The originators will usually be the families and people who have been injured who have come together to organize head-injury societies, and they will have to mobilize every source of help that they can. Good luck to them!

Organizing a head-injury service requires commitment from:
the head injured
their families
concerned professionals
the public
politicians

12 Suggestions for further reading

For the non-specialist, non-medical reader

Bryant, Beverley (1992) *In search of wings: A journey back from traumatic brain injury*. Wings Press, South Paris, Maine

Weiss, L., Thatch, D., and Thatch, J. with Gray, L. (1983). *I wasn't finished with life*. E. Hart Press, Dallas, Texas.

For the non-specialist medical or paramedical reader

Levin, H. S., Eisenberg, H. M., and Benton, A. L. (ed) (1989) *Mild head injury*. Oxford University Press, New York.

Lezak, Muriel, D. (ed) (1989) *Assessment of the Behavioural consequences of head injury*. Alan R. Liss, New York.

Ponsford, Jennie (1995) *Traumatic brain injury : Rehabilitation for everyday adaptive living*. Lawrence Erlbaum Associates, East Sussex

For the specialist medical or paramedical reader

Brooks, N. (ed) (1984) *Closed head injury: psychological, social, and family consequences*. Oxford University Press, New York.

Richardson, John T. E. (1990) *Clinical and neuropsychological aspects of closed head injury*. Taylor & Francis, London

Appendix A: Glossary

Acceleration injury. Damage to the brain caused by sudden movement, when the soft brain is distorted and torn.

Agnosia. Loss of the ability to know the meaning of significance of things. It can affect our interpretation of what we see or hear, the parts of the body, or taste and smell.

Agraphia. Total (dysgraphia partial) loss of the ability to express ourselves in writing.

Alexia. Total (dyslexia partial) loss of our ability to read which can affect written language, symbols, or music scores.

Amnesia. Loss of the ability to remember things done or experienced (see also retrograde, pre-traumatic, and post traumatic amnesia).

Anarthria. Total (dysarthria partial) loss of speech due to impaired function of the larynx and throat. The use of language to express oneself may or may not be normal.

Anosmia. Loss of the sense of smell and fine taste.

Anticonvulsants. Medication to control epilepsy.

Aphasia. Total (dysphasia partial) loss of the ability to make oneself understood (expressive dysphasia), or to understand others (receptive dysphasia), by the use of language. It can affect the use of speech, writing, listening or reading, and sign language.

Anoxia. Lack of oxygen, in this context for the brain cells.

Apraxia. Total (dyspraxia partial) loss of the ability to carry out purposeful movements, though one still has the ability to move and be aware of movement.

Ataxia. Impaired coordination of movement.

Blood clots. See haematoma.

Brain stem. The deep central part of the brain, connecting the cerebral hemispheres with the spinal cord. It contains centres for the maintenance of consciousness, the control of movement and balance, and of vital organs as the heart and lungs.

Burr hole. A hole drilled through the skull, often needed to measure and control intracranial pressure.

Central nervous system (CNS). The brain and spinal cord.

Cerebellum. Part of the brain located at its base and behind the brain stem. It is important for the control of movement.

CAT Scan (CT Scan). Computerized axial tomography, an X-ray procedure which gives a picture of soft tissue, especially of the brain, as well as of bone.

Cerebral cortex. The folded ridged grey matter on the surface of the cerebral hemispheres.

Cerebral hemispheres. The two side-by-side halves of the cerebrum, the main part of the brain.

Cerebral oedema. Swelling of the brain—see Oedema.

Cerebrospinal fluid (CSF). The clear colourless fluid in the ventricles of the brain and the spaces round it and the spinal cord.

Cerebrum. The main part of the brain which sits in the upper part of the skull cavity, consisting principally of the two cerebral hemispheres.

Chorea. Involuntary movements which occur in some cases after head injury.

Closed head injury. Damage to the brain when there has not been a wound or penetrating injury.

Coma. A state of altered consciousness, when the person is not reacting normally to stimuli.

Coma score. A way of recording the depth of coma, on a scale from deep unconsciousness with no reaction to any sort of stimulus, through response only to pain, later to confused response to speech and then to normal function. Commonly used is the Glasgow Coma score, on a 3 to 15 point scale.

Compound fracture. A facture of the skull with a wound over it.

Concussion. A mild head injury, with temporary disturbance of brain function, usually but not always with a short loss of consciousness; it may have persisting effects.

Contusion. Bruising, in this context usually of the brain.

Cough reflex. The automatic cough which clears the throat and lungs of secretions in the awake person, but which is absent when a patient is unconscious so that lung function is impaired and infection occurs.

Cranium. The skull.

Critical Care. See Intensive Care.

CSF rhinorrhoea. Cerebrospinal fluid leaking into the nose from a fracture in its roof.

Diplopia. Double vision.

Dura mater. The tough membrane lying between the brain and the bone of the skull.

Dysarthria. See Anarthria.

Dysgraphia. See Agraphia.

Dyslexia. See Alexia.

Dysphasia. See Aphasia.

Dyspraxia. See Apraxia.

Electroencephalogram (EEG). A recording of the electrical activity of the brain, taken from electrodes placed on the scalp. Used in the early stages to assess damage and later in the diagnosis of post-traumatic epilepsy.

Evoked potentials (Somatosensory evoked potentials, SEPs). Recordings of the EEG changes produced by stimulating a nerve in the arm or by sound; the speed of the response and its character can indicate the extent of damage to the brain.

Extradural. Between the dura mater and the skull, usually used to describe a clot of blood forming there.

Frontal lobe. The front third of each cerebral hemisphere; damage here affects the organization of many of the other areas of the brain, and has a particular effect on a person's behaviour and insight into their condition.

Gastrostomy. Inserting a feeding tube directly into the stomach through the abdominal wall; done either by an open operation or through a telescope passed down the throat into the stomach. Used for long term nutrition.

Haematoma. A collection or clot of blood, which may be within the brain or pressing on it from outside.

Haemorrhage. Bleeding.

Hemianopia. Loss of sight in one half of the field of vision, affecting both eyes: due to damage to nerves within the skull or to the occipital lobes of the brain.

Hemineglect. Loss of attention to things on one side of the body; usually due to damage to the parietal lobe of the brain on the opposite side.

Hemeplegia. Paralysis (hemiparesis weakness) of one side of the body, due either to damage to the opposite side of the brain, or in severe injuries to the brainstem.

Hydrocephalus. Accumulation of fluid in the ventricles of the brain, causing symptoms from increase of pressure. Occasionally a late complication of head injury.

Infarct. An area of brain in which the cells have died because of a loss of blood supply.

Intensive care. A hospital department having the means to observe an injured person closely and continually, using complex monitoring equipment, and to respond immediately with any treatment which becomes necessary.

Intracerebral. Within the substance of the brain, in this context usually describing a clot of blood present there.

Intracranial pressure. The pressure inside the skull. Increased by blood clots, brain contusion and oedema it is a critical factor in survival after head injury; measurement and control is a vital part of treatment.

Mild head injury. A head injury from which the majority of people recover rapidly and completely, though in a small percentage there are persisting problems.

MR Scan (Magnetic Resonance Scan). A procedure which like the CT scan gives a picture of the soft tissue of the brain, but which uses a strong magnetic field and radio waves rather than X-rays.

Nasogastric tube. A fine tube passed down to the stomach through the mouth or nose, so that liquid food can be given before normal swallowing is possible.

Neuron. A nerve cell.

Occipital lobe. The back part of each cerebral hemisphere. Damage on one side may result in hemianopia, and can affect how we understand things that are seen, with dyslexia.

Oedema. Excess fluid accumulating in the brain, due to injury. An important factor in increase of intracranial pressure.

Open head injury. A head injury in which there is a wound to the brain which communicates with the outside.

Paramedics. People trained in the techniques of urgent treatment at the scene of the accident and of transport to hospital care.

Parietal lobe. The upper middle part of each cerebral hemisphere. Damage to various parts of the lobe affects movement, speech, sensation, and awareness of the world around.

Penetrating injury. An injury in which there is a wound which reaches the brain.

Photophobia. Abnormal sensitivity of the eyes to light.

Post-traumatic amnesia (PTA). Loss of memory for events immediately following a head injury, which may continue when the person has regained consciousness. Sometimes islands of memory occur early or late in the amnesia but the amnesia is not said to end until recall becomes continuous.

Post-traumatic epilepsy. Epileptic seizures occurring due brain damage in a head injury; may be of several types.

Pre-traumatic amnesia. See Retrograde amnesia.

Retrograde amnesia. Loss of memory for events occurring for a period before the head injury.

Second accident. Occurring typically in a traffic accident when the already injured person is thrown out of the vehicle and suffers further damage.

Second injury. The damage which is done to the brain by lack of oxygen and low blood pressure in the time between the accident and the arrival of expert care.

Second injury syndrome. The catastrophic deterioration which may occur when a second head injury occurs within a week or two of the first; most often recognized after milder injuries in sport.

Spastic paralysis. Absence of voluntary movement, but with the muscles contracting spontaneously and resisting any attempt to move the limb.

Subdural. Inside the dura mater; usually referring to a clot of blood developing between the dura and the brain.

Temporal lobe. A lobe of the brain situated below the parietal lobe. The left lobe is important in speech and the right in perception of space and form, and both sides are concerned with recent memory. Their position makes them liable to damage in acceleration injuries.

Third injury. The damage done to the brain by complications such as haematomas, usually occurring in the first two days after the accident.

Tracheo(s)tomy. Making an opening in the windpipe to allow easy breathing, used when the injured person is likely to be unconscious for a long period.

Vault. The rounded upper part of the skull, in distinction to the base of the skull.

Ventilator. The mechanical device used to take over breathing in the deeply unconscious patient.

Ventricles. The four cavities inside the brain. Cerebrospinal fluid is formed in them and flows out into the spaces outside the brain; obstruction to this flow causes hydrocephalus.

Vocational rehabilitation. Preparing for the return to work.

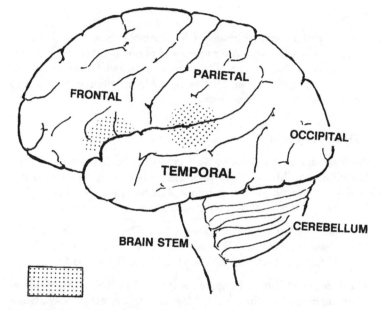

AREAS ON THE LEFT SIDE OF
THE BRAIN CONCERNED WITH SPEECH

Appendix B: Contacts for family support groups

Contact persons and addresses of local support groups are liable to change frequently and so the address and phone number of the parent association has been given. The parent organization will be able to provide information about what is available in different areas in the country and an up-to-date contact.

INTERNATIONAL

An international brain injury association has been formed since the first edition of this book was published. They proposed to publish a National Directory of Brain Injury Rehabilitation Services in late June, 1997. For information on this, contact

Monique J. Marino, Publications Chief Operating Officer, 1776 Massachusetts Avenue, N.W., Suite 100, Washington, D.C. 20036-1904, U.S.A. Phone: (202) 296 6443. Fax: (202) 296 8850

The Director of Family Programs is Alice Demichelis, International Brain Injury Association, 1776 Massachusetts Avenue, N.W., Suite 105, Washington, D.C. 20036-1904, U.S.A. Phone: (202) 835 0580. Fax: (202) 835 0584

GREAT BRITAIN

Ian Garrow O.B.E., Executive Director,
Headway, National Head Injuries Association, 7 King Edward Court, King Edward Street, Nottingham, NG1 1EW, UK. Phone: (115) 924 0800. Fax: (115) 924 0432

UNITED STATES OF AMERICA

National Head Injury Foundation (Inc), 333 Turnpike Road, Southborough, MA 01772, USA. Phone: (508) 485–9950 Family Help Line: Phone: (508) 485 9950

AUSTRALIA

The Head Injury Council of Australia (HICOA), PO Box 304, Port Melbourne 3207, Australia. Phone: (03) 696–1388

This body represents all state head-injury organizations, and supplied the following addresses of associated state groups:

Kel Buchanan, Vice President HICOA, Administrator, Head-Injury Society of Western Australia, PO Box 298, Applecross 6154, Australia. Phone: (09) 3306370

Alana Clohesy, Director, Headway New South Wales, PO Box 424, Burwood 2134, Australia. Phone: (02) 7472866

Alwyn Ricci, President, Headway Queensland, 38 Flower Street, Nundah 4012, Australia. Phone: (07) 2667664

Frank Quigley, President, Head-Injury Society of South Australia, PO Box 20, Stepney 5069, Australia. Phone: (08) 2646275

NEW ZEALAND

Harley Pope, Director, Brain Injury Association, 207 Manakau Road, Epsom, Auckland 3. Phone: (09) 623 1813

Head Injury Society of New Zealand, P.O. Box 12-245, Wellington. Phone: (04) 472 0977

Index